CARB CYCLING

The Recipe and Diet Book

2nd Edition

Jesse Morgan

<u>CONTENTS</u>

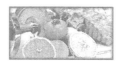

CHAPTER 1

Why you should purchase and read this book

Carb cycling is a relatively simple concept that offers real world results. This is probably not the first book you've read on dieting so you know what is out there. The list is endless; carb free diets, high protein diets, paleo diets. Each diet has its benefits and shortcomings. Carb Cycling allows you to continue to enjoy the foods you like while still reducing weight and/or body fat.

This diet is used by professional body builders, athletes and regular everyday people that want to lose fat, get healthy and look good.

What this book will do for YOU

1. Explain the concepts of carbohydrate cycling and why this diet can and will work if you follow it.

2. Help you prepare properly so you can give yourself a fighting chance.

3. Provide a listing of foods you should and should not eat.

4. Deliver a simple to follow step by step action plan.

5. Offer recipes for meals that fit the diet, use healthy ingredients and are easy to prepare.

6. Provide a journal you can use to track your progress.

Give me one hour of your time and you will have a good understanding of the carbohydrate cycling diet. Then it is up to you to decide if you are ready for the change. I am not a doctor, nutritionist or weight loss guru, I am just like you, someone that is interested in finding the best way to maintain a healthy weight, stay fit and live long. I have done the work for you of collecting the best information from across the web and from various diet books to help you make an informed decision on whether this diet is right for you or not.

I am confident you will walk away with a much better understanding of carbohydrate cycling and of the foods you should and shouldn't eat. I think that information is well worth the price of this book and hope you will agree when you have finished reading it.

You can download a printable copy of the weekly diet journal and a detailed listing of the ingredients used in the recipes along with the nutritional details at www.carbcycle.net.

If you found at least some value in this book, whether its the nutrition information, diet plan, recipes, journal or a combination of any or all, please write a review on Amazon.com. Postive 4 & 5 star reviews really help thank you ! - Jesse..

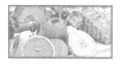

CHAPTER 2

Why Carb Cycling?

The great thing about carbohydrate cycling is that you really don't have to change the foods you are used to eating, just the timing of when you eat those foods. Experts say it takes at least 30 days to form a habit, you need to give this program at least 30 days if you expect to see results. Once you break through that point, this method of eating should become second nature to you.

If you have ever tried a low-carb or no-carb diet you are probably familiar with the effects on your body like cravings, lack of energy and inability to think clearly. This is because your body has grown accustomed to the levels of sugar in your normal diet.

Carb Cycling has been used by body builders for years to help drop their percentage of fat to low single digits. In the past 5 years this diet has hit the mainstream as a better alternative to the low carbohydrate diets.

The Science behind Carb Cycling

This section is important even if you are not an athlete, it will give you a better understanding of how your body uses the food

you eat for fuel. When you eat carbohyd
system converts them to glucose.

The glucose will be processed by the
body in one of the following three ways:

1. Meet immediate demands for
   energy.

2. Restore glycogen levels in your liver and your
   muscles.

3. Convert to fat cells and store for later use (hopefully).

Glycogen is stored by the body and then later used to generate
energy. Endurance athletes like marathoners log long hours
of training in advance of their event. One of the byproducts of
this training is an increase in their ability to store glycogen for
later use. The body uses four primary sources of fuel for energy;
glycogen, glucose, fat and finally protein from muscle.

Glycogen is the most efficient form of fuel for your body
followed by glucose from food you have recently consumed.
Athletes will often consume performance gels while they are
working out. These gels are primarily sugar and can quickly be
converted by the body to energy.

Aerobic vs. anaerobic training

When you workout, your level of effort determines which
energy systems are used as the main source of fuel. The primary
difference is oxygen. In an aerobic workout, your oxygen intake
matches or exceeds the needs of your muscles. This allows your

muscles to burn a combination of glycogen, carbohydrates and fat for energy. As you increase your intensity, your muscles need more oxygen and rely primarily on glycogen stores and available carbohydrates.

You may have read that aerobic training burns more fat since you are working out at a slower pace. It is true that your body can convert a higher percentage of fat to energy during aerobic workouts, however you still burn more calories and in turn more fat when working out with a mix of aerobic and anaerobic efforts. Interval training is a great way to improve any workout and burn more calories. For example, if you are jogging on a treadmill, go easy for 3 minutes and then increase the intensity and push your limits for 30 seconds, repeat this 10 times for a great session. You could do the same thing with a jog around the neighborhood, bike ride or other workout.

Carb Cycling - The Big Picture

1. Alternate high and low carbohydrate days.

2. Eat 5 to 6 smaller meals a day.

3. Stay away from simple carbohydrates and try to reduce sugar intake.

4. Make sure to schedule your workouts on high carbohydrate days.

5. Take a reward day once a week and eat whatever you want.

Your workout effort will be based on your current ability. Ideally you should shoot for at least three aerobic and one strength training workouts per week. If you are not working out at all you can start slow and build up, if you have a strong workout schedule, you can continue what you are doing and just incorporate in the diet. Try to avoid going "all out" on your first workout, you will just end up tired and sore.

Macro-nutrients required to sustain life

Protein

You need protein each day to function properly. Your body breaks down proteins into amino acids that are used to power your systems. The protein is used to build and repair tissues, create hormones, enzymes and other body chemicals. It is a critical building block for muscles, bones, skin and even blood.

If you search for protein on the web you will find a substantial amount of conflicting information on how much protein you need on a daily basis. Keep it simple, have some protein with each meal. This was a big change for me, my diet used to be about 80% carbohydrates.

Carbohydrates

The primary source of energy for your body. Every cell in your body uses glucose (a form of sugar) for energy. Once your body digests carbohydrates the glucose that is produced must be used immediately to generate energy or be stored in the liver or your muscles as glycogen. Once the glycogen reserves are full, the only choice left is to store those sugars as fat. There in lies the problem when you eat too many carbohydrates or eat them late in the day when your energy requirements are usually low.

Big pasta dinner at 7pm followed by a couples of hours on the couch watching Breaking Bad and Mad Men. You can pretty much bet most of that glucose is going to convert right over to fat cells. Try to eat carbohydrates earlier in the day if possible and avoid things like rice, pasta and potatoes at dinner.

Healthy Fats

The big trend in dieting for years was the low-fat diet. The food industry quickly responded with low-fat versions of just about every processed food available. The problem is the fat was replaced with sodium, sugar and loads of chemicals. Healthy fats include monounsaturated and polyunsaturated fats, you can find a listing of the foods that fall into these two groups in the nutrition 101 chapter.

The fats to stay away from are saturated and trans fat which include items like butter, cheese, donuts, packaged snack food and fried foods. I know that sounds like all the good stuff but stick with me it is not all bad.

Researchers at Genesis Prevention Center at University Hospital in South Manchester, England, found that restricting carbohydrates two days per week may be a better dietary approach than a standard, daily calorie-restricted diet for preventing breast cancer and other diseases, but they said further study is needed.

"Weight loss and reduced insulin levels are required for breast cancer prevention, but [these levels] are difficult to achieve and maintain with conventional dietary approaches," said Michelle Harvie, Ph.D., SRD, a research dietician at the Genesis Prevention Center, who presented the findings at the 2011 CTRC-AACR San Antonio Breast Cancer Symposium, held Dec. 6-10, 2011.

Why does Carb Cycling work?

1. You are still eating sufficient quantities of the three macro-nutrients (fat, protein & carbs).

2. You don't have to change your lifestyle to maintain your diet.

3. The food you are eating is healthy, unprocessed and it even tastes good.

4. You won't find yourself craving foods as much as you would on other diets.

5. You can incorporate this diet into your family meals with only minimal changes.

One important note, you may find that your weight climbs and decreases a bit more than on other diets, your goal is weight loss over the course of the diet. Think of it like you would your retirement savings. If you look at it everyday, you will lose your mind. Check in once a week and see how you are progressing.

Want more information on good and bad calories? Check out Cathy Wilson's book, *Good vs. Bad Calories 101* on Amazon. com.

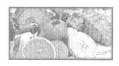

CHAPTER 3

Prepare and You Will Succeed

The key to succeeding at any new endeavor is to clearly understand what you are going to do, why you want or need to do it and how you will accomplish your goal.

Preparation

- Review the shopping list and glycemic index charts to get an idea of the foods you should and shouldn't be eating.

- Review the menu options and give thought to the types of food you will need to have in the house. One of the benefits of this diet is you don't have to completely change the foods you are accustomed to, that is provided you don't live on fried foods and prepared snack foods.

- Review the workout chapter and determine your exercise plan. You can follow one of the workouts in this book or use a workout program from another book or website. The program itself is not that critical, just find something that you will stick with.

- Keep track of your progress. If you bought the paperback version of this book, you have a 26 week journal. If you purchased the e-book version, you can download a printable journal at www.controlyourday.net/carbcycle.

- Sign up for a free account at www.myfitnesspal.com. This is a great tool that you can use from a web browser, your smart-phone or your tablet. The site has thousands of foods with all of the nutritional information. You can keep track of what you eat and easily see how many calories you are consuming as well as the counts of macro nutrients (protein, carbohydrates and fats).

- Determine your daily calories, MyFitnessPal will do this for you once you enter in your information and weight loss goals. You can also use the chart below from the Institute of Medicine. The numbers below are a bit high if you want to lose weight. When I put my information into MyFitnessPal it suggested 1,650 calories per day to hit my weight loss goals.

Gender	Age	Sedentary	Moderately Active	Active
Female	14-18	1,800	2,000	2,400
	19-30	2,000	2,000-2,200	2,400
	31-50	1,800	2,000	2,200
	51+	1,600	1,800	2,000-2,200
Male	14-18	2,200	2,400-2,800	2,800-3,200
	19-30	2,400	2,600-2,800	3,000
	31-50	2,200	2,400-2,600	2,800-3,000
	51+	2,000	2,200-2,400	2,400-2,800

The calorie estimates in the chart are from the Institute of Medicine

Dietary Reference Intakes macro-nutrients report, 2002.

Sedentary is a lifestyle that includes only light physical activity related to daily life.

Moderately Active is a lifestyle that includes physical activity (exercise or sports) of at least 2 to 3 hours.

Active is a lifestyle that includes 3 to 6 hours or more of exercise or sports activity a week.

Use MyFitnessPal to monitor your calories and your allocation of carbs, protein and fats. Don't worry too much about the calories as long as you are in the correct range you are fine. They key is not to be way off the baseline. For example if you are supposed to eat 2,200 calories a day and on your low carb days you only eat 1,500 calories, you need to eat more as your body will begin to slow your metabolism to match the caloric intake. Same goes the other way, if you are 500 calories over your baseline everyday you will end up gaining weight.

Once you determine your calories per day, you can calculate the # of grams of protein, fat and carbs by using the following per-centages. MyFitnessPal will show you the percentage of calories for each macro-nutrient as you make entries to the food log. To keep this simple, we will use a daily allowance of 2000 calories.

First calculate the # of calories for each macro nutrient

Low-Carb Day

20% of calories from Carbs = 400 calories
50% of calories from Protein = 1000 calories
30% of calories from Fats = 600 calories

High-Carb Day

45% of calories from Carbs = 900 calories
40% of calories from Protein = 800 calories
15% of calories from Fats = 300 calories

Next convert those calories into grams, for protein and carbs divide calories by 4, for fat divide by 9. Here is what that would look like for the 2,000 calorie diet.

Low-Carb Day

20% of calories from Carbs = 100 grams
50% of calories from Protein = 250 grams
30% of calories from Fats = 67 grams

High-Carb Day

45% of calories from Carbs = 225 grams calories
40% of calories from Protein = 200 grams
15% of calories from Fats = 33 calories

Here it is in one straight line equation for the low carb day.

$2000 \times .20 / 4 = 100$ grams carbs

$2000 \times .50 / 4 = 250$ grams protein

2000 x .30 / 9 = 67 grams fat

That may have been a bit confusing. If you use MyFitnessPal, it will handle all of the calculations for you and just show you the percentages of each macro-nutrient consumed. If you are a numbers or detail person and you want to get more information on these calculation, go to www.caloriesperhour.com, you will find a number of different nutrition calculators you can use.

Make the commitment to yourself to do this for at least 30 days so you can give the diet a chance to work and see the results for yourself. If you fail, it is OK, get up, dust yourself off and start over again. Babe Ruth has the record for the third highest home run record in baseball, did you know that for a decade he held the record for the highest strikeouts as well. When asked about it he said: "Every strike brings me closer to my next home run".

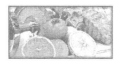

CHAPTER 4

The Benefits of Exercise

If you want to lose weight and fat you need to combine a good diet with a regular exercise plan. I am not a doctor, coach or trainer, discuss any new exercise plans with your doctor or trainer before starting them.

I am now an avid exerciser, but that was not always the case. In my mid 30's I was overweight and unhealthy. I started my journey by deciding to run a marathon. I was never a big runner, so I was starting from zero. I found a great training book that guided me through the whole process titled "The Non-Runner's Marathon Trainer, it is available on Amazon.com. I finished my first marathon in 4:50 minutes and ran two more with a best time of 4:18 minutes. I then moved on to mountain biking and road cycling and added in the Beachbody training programs.

My lifestyle is completely different today, I eat healthy, get a good nights rest, keep my stress levels under control and workout at least 4 to 5 times per week. My point is, you need to start somewhere, and if you have already started, then its time to step it up a notch. You only get one chance on the planet, you might as well make the best of it.

If you have no exercise routine today, then you may want to start out making just some small changes to your daily routine. For example taking the stairs instead of the elevator, taking a walk before work or at lunch. If you have access to a gym spend at least 30 to 40 minutes on your high carbohydrate days on a treadmill, stepper or elliptical. You will not see the same level of results, but you need to start somewhere. Resist the temptation to "crush it" the first day in the gym, you don't want to start off feeling miserable and sore or worse end up with an injury that limits your ability to exercise.

Here are a few articles to get you started on you started on the right foot:

http://www.webmd.com/fitness-exercise/guide/fitness-
    beginners-guide

http://www.mayoclinic.com/health/fitness/HQ00171

http://health.howstuffworks.com/wellness/diet-fitness/
    exercise/starting-an-exercise-program.htm

The key to success is to keep putting in the effort. Do some form of exercise on each of your high-carb days. Even if you have to break it up during the day, its still better than no exercise at all. Ideally you want to exercise for at least 30 minutes, you want to get your heart rate up and work up a sweat. I realize that may not be realistic in the beginning, just start and do what you can.

Think about how many hours a day you spend sitting. Does this sound like your day? Wake up, shower and get dressed, sit down for breakfast, drive to work, sit down at your desk, sit down at lunch, sit down at your desk, drive home, sit down for dinner, sit down to watch some TV, head to bed.

A few simple changes and you can start burning extra calories. When you wake up in the morning take 5 or 10 minutes to stretch or do some yoga. Can you ride a bike to work or maybe park a bit further out in the parking lot (provided its safe)? Can you take the stairs instead of the elevator? Any possibility to stand up for part of your day with a raised desk or even just when you are meeting with others? How about a walk around the building at lunch time?

If you are a stay-at-home mom or dad. You probably spend more time on your feet, running errands, doing laundry, cleaning house. Can you block out a few 15 or 20 minute segments for a few quick workouts? Maybe a brisk walk around the block or ten minutes going up and down the stairs? If you put some effort into it, you can find ways to incorporate some level of exercise into your daily routine.

If you need some help getting motivated, checkout the Fitbit Flex Wireless Activity wristband. It keeps track of your steps and activity throughout the day. You can track your activity on-line and even compete against friends and other users.

Casual Exerciser

You might have a gym membership that gets occasional use or maybe you get out a few days a week for a walk, light run or bike ride. You are not challenging your body which means you are not building any new muscle, if you are older than 40 you are losing muscle each year. Think about a skill, activity or hobby that you have done for a long period of time. In the beginning, it may have been challenging, but now after years of practice you can do it with your eyes closed. This is the way your body works with exercise. If you go out and walk the same 3 mile loop 3 times a week, your body acclimates itself to that workout and will no longer challenged by it.

You need to change up your workout routines and challenge your body. The best way to do that is with interval training. Consider the daily walk or jog, instead of just going out and exercising at the same pace, push yourself for short periods, you could use mailboxes or driveways as your markers to start and stop your intervals. You could change from a walk to a jog every third mailbox or if you are not ready for that just pick up your walking pace.

Schedule your workouts for your high-carb days, you can work out more often than that if you want to. Make sure to mix in at least one strength training workout a week, two would be ideal. If you are in decent shape and want to take your fitness to a new level check out the Beachbody programs at www.beachbody.com. You have probably seen their infomercials on Saturday or Sunday morning on the TV. The programs work. I've been through P90x, Insanity and now T25.

P90x provides the best overall workout with a combination of weights, cardio and stretch. You can do all the workouts in your home, garage or local gym, all you need is a few dumbbells and a pull-up bar. The workouts run about 1 hour.

Insanity is tough, it is 40 to 80 minutes of non-stop impact training. If you are in great shape, these routines could take you to the next level.

Their latest program is T25. This is a focused 25 minute workout 5 days a week. I recently started this routine and absolutely love it. I can always find 25 minutes to workout and it requires nothing but a 4x6 area and a decent pair of sneakers.

If video workouts are not your gig, check out your local gym to see what classes they have. Check out a spin class, body pump or cross training session. These are all great workouts, you will put in a stronger effort when you are part of a class.

Finally here are a few websites that offer simple workout programs:

http://www.shape.com/fitness/workouts/interval-training-short-workouts-really-pay

http://sportsmedicine.about.com/od/tipsandtricks/a/Intervals.htm

And finally an article from the New York Times talking about the benefits of interval training. Here is a quote from the article.

A 2005 study published in the Journal of Applied Physiology found that after just two weeks of interval training, six of the eight college-age men and women doubled their endurance, or the amount of time they could ride a bicycle at moderate intensity before exhaustion.

http://tinyurl.com/nytimesworkout

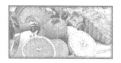

CHAPTER 5

Nutrition 101 - Building a New Shopping List

This chapter starts with the positive and then turns to the dark side to cover the foods and additives you should stay away from. Your goal should be to lose weight, lose fat and improve your health. In order to do that you need to be well educated about the food you put into your body.

This list provides a great starting point for you to use to shop for your new eating lifestyle. You can expand the list just make sure you are adding healthy items to the list in the correct categories.

Protein Sources	Carbs - Misc.	Carbs - Fruit	Vegetables	Fats
Eggs	Beans/Legumes	Apple	Asparagus	Avocado
Egg Whites	Brown Rice	Apricot	Broccoli	Coconut Oil
Skim Milk	Corn	Banana	Carrots	Flax Seed Oil
Low Fat Yogurt	Oats	Berry	Celery	Grass Fed Butter
Cottage Cheese (1% Fat)	Peas	Grape	Cucumbers	Macadamia Nut
Protein Powder	Popcorn	Kiwi	Green Beans	*Nut Butter
Tuna	Potatoes	Melon	Onions	Olive Oil
Salmon	Quinoa	Orange	Peppers	*Raw nuts
Shelfish	Sweet Potatos	Peach	Radishes	Walnut Oil
Chicken (skinless-white)	Whole Grain Bread	Pear	Spinach	

Lean Beef	Whole Grain Pasta	Pineapple		* No Peanuts
Turkey (skinless-white)	Wild Rice	Plum		

My Go To Food List

This is a great list of healthy fast food options. Most of the items below can be prepared with just a microwave, single pot/pan or grill. Everything you see listed below can be found at a local warehouse club like BJ's or Costco. If you are not a member of one of the warehouse clubs, I would recommend you sign up. It will make your shopping and food preparation easier and cheaper.

- Pre-cooked chicken sausage
- Pre-cooked chicken strips
- Turkey Burgers
- Avocados
- Mixed Nuts
- Eggs
- Egg Whites
- Part-Skim low fat mozzarella cheese
- Muscle Milk Whey Protein
- Frozen mixed vegetables
- Frozen Blueberries (wild or organic or both)
- Red Grapefruit single serve cups
- Greek Yogurt
- Almond Butter

If you buy the cheese at a wholesale club it will be more than you can consume before the opened product expires. Pack the cheese into sandwich or quart size zip-lock bags and place them in the freezer. Write the freeze date on each bag. When you open the bag you can write the date opened on the bag as well. This way you will know how long it has been sitting in your refrigerator. You should use the refrigerated cheese within 7 to 10 days. Sargento (maker of cheese) suggests freezing for no more than 2 months.

The one item on the list above that is questionable is Whey Protein. It is not a natural food source, it is highly processed. Whey Protein does provide a great way to add protein to your diet with minimal calories or fat, but you need to recognize it has some negative attributes.

The No Fly Zone (Stay away from these foods)

If you want to succeed with your diet, you need to get serious about the foods you include in your diet. Here is the New Zealand Medical Journal's list of non-essential, energy dense, nutritionally deficient foods. I am sure you noticed alcohol is #1 on the list, don't panic this list is in alphabetical order.

1. Alcoholic drinks
2. Biscuits (cookies)
3. Butter, lard, dripping or similar fat (used as a spread or in baking/cooking etc.)
4. Cakes
5. Chocolate
6. Coconut cream
7. Condensed milk
8. Cordial
9. Corn chips
10. Cream (including creme fraiche)

11. Crisps (including vegetable crisps)
12. Desserts/puddings
13. Doughnuts
14. Drinking Chocolate, Milo etc.
15. Energy drinks
16. Flavored milk/milkshakes
17. Fruit tinned in syrup
18. Fried food
19. Frozen yogurt
20. Fruit juice (except tomato juice and unsweetened blackcurrant juice)
21. Glucose
22. High fat crackers
23. Honey
24. Hot chips
25. Ice cream
26. Jam
27. Marmalade
28. Mayonnaise
29. Muesli bars
30. Muffins
31. Nuts roasted in fat or oil
32. Pastries
33. Pies
34. Popcorn with butter or oil
35. Quiches
36. Reduced cream
37. Regular luncheon sausage

38. Regular powdered drinks
39. Regular salami
40. Regular sausages
41. Regular soft drinks
42. Fruit roll-ups
43. Sour cream
44. Sugar (added to anything including drinks, baking, cooking etc.)
45. Sweets/lollies
46. Syrups such as golden syrup, treacle, maple syrup
47. Toasted muesli and any other breakfast cereal with more than 15g sugar per 100g cereal
48. Whole milk
49. Yogurt type products with more than 15g of sugar

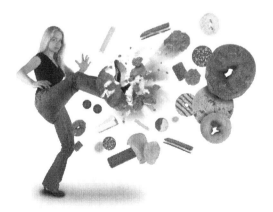

Try to reduce the sugar you consume each day

If you use MyFitnessPal you can easily see how many grams of sugar you are eating a day. The American Heart Association suggests the maximum amount of added sugars you should eat per day is 37.5 grams for men and 25 grams per women. I think those numbers are just about impossible to attain. An average cup of fruit yogurt usually has about 21 grams of sugar. You really need to look at the nutritional

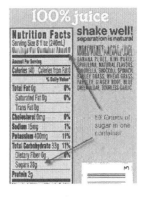

labels on the food you eat if you want to make a dent in your sugar consumption. I stopped putting sugar in my coffee, stopped using ketchup (contains corn syrup) and changed to Greek yogurt.

Check the labels sugar has many names including; agave nectar, barley malt syrup, corn sweetener, corn syrup, dextrin, dextrose, fructose, glucose, high fructose corn syrup, honey, lactose, maltodextrin, malt syrup, molasses, saccharose, sorghum, sucrose and xylose.

Reducing sugar intake is not a key component of the Carb Cycling diet but it is something that will help you to reduce weight and improve your health.

This popular juice is sold in a container that appears to be designed for one serving. You might grab this thinking it is a healthy choice to get your day started. Think again. If you drink the 16 ounce container you have just consumed 280 calories, almost no protein and a whopping 56 grams of sugar which is more than the American Heart Association recommends for the entire day. Remember if your body is unable to immediately burn sugar to generate energy it has to be converted to fat.

Check out Peggy Annear's new book "Sugar Free Recipes: Low Carb Low Sugar Recipes on a Sugar Smart Diet. The Savvy No Sugar Diet Guide & Cookbook" on amazon.com for some great recipes.

Watch out for high levels of Sodium

The American Heart Association recommends limiting your sodium intake to less than 2,000 milligrams per day. Eating canned foods, frozen meals and restaurant meals can easily take you above the limits.

Nutrition Facts

Serving Size: 1 cup (244g)

Amount Per Serving

Calories 129	Calories from Fat 81
	% Daily Value*
Total Fat 8.98 g	14%
Saturated Fat 2.44 g	12%
Trans Fat	
Cholesterol 2.44 mg	1%
Sodium 890.84 mg	37%
Potassium 100.04 mg	3%

This label is from a can of creamy mushroom soup. One serving contains almost half of the daily recommended sodium. Add in a frozen meal for lunch and a take out dinner and you will easily exceed the 2,000mg level.

Hydrogenated and Partially Hydrogenated oils are the devil

Check your labels folks if you see hydrogenated or partially hydrogenated fat listed as an ingredient, walk away. These fats, also called trans fats, raise your bad (LDL) cholesterol and lower your good (HDL) cholesterol levels. They will increase your risk 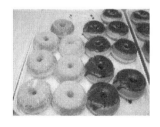 of heart disease and stroke. These fats cause comparatively more weight gain than a similar diet with monounsaturated fats, they are also associated with atherosclerosis and inflammation.

MSG is Everywhere

Monosodium Glutomate (MSG) is a flavor enhancer widely known as an addition to Chinese food. It can be found in chips, soups, sauces and just about every fast food restaurant on the planet. The FDA claims there are no adverse health concerns with MSG, but if you search around the web you will find an endless stream of information on the negative effects of MSG on the body. Estimates say that as many as 40% of the population have an intolerance for MSG. Reactions to MSG include numbness, burning sensation, headache, nausea, chest pain, rapid heartbeat and other symptoms. Obesity, eye damage and depression have been linked to regular consumption of MSG.

Checking your ingredients label for MSG is not enough. Look for any of these words in the ingredients list, they all contain MSG.

- Aspartame
- Autolyzed
- Caseinate
- Gelatin
- Glutamate
- Glutamic Acid
- Hydrolyzed
- Plant Protein
- Textured Protein

There are many more ingredients that contain MSG. Search for "Ingredients with MSG" on the web and you will find millions of pages that provide detailed lists. Unfortunately it is just about impossible to completely remove MSG from your diet, but at least if you know what to look for you can reduce the amount you do consume.

Dirty Dozen - 12 Fruits & Veggies with the most pesticides

Just when you thought you were safe by focusing on whole foods, there is some bad news when it comes to conventionally (non-organic) grown fruits and vegetables. The 12 listed below should be purchased organically to reduce your intake of harmful pesticides.

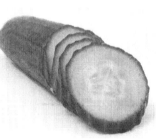

1. Apples
2. Celery
3. Cherry Tomatoes
4. Cucumbers
5. Grapes
6. Hot Peppers
7. Nectarines (imported)
8. Peaches
9. Potatoes
10. Spinach
11. Strawberries
12. Sweet bell peppers

The news is not all bad, there are many fruits and vegetables that are grown conventionally that are safe to eat.

Clean 15

1. Asparagus
2. Avocados
3. Cabbage
4. Cantaloupe
5. Sweet corn
6. Eggplant
7. Grapefruit
8. Kiwi
9. Mangoes
10. Mushrooms
11. Onions
12. Papayas
13. Pineapples
14. Sweet peas
15. Sweet potatoes

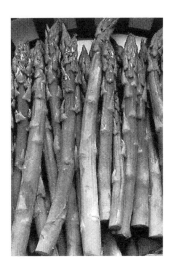

My goal for this chapter was to provide some insight on the types of food that will help you achieve your goals and the foods that you should stay away from if you want to maintain a healthy body. Here is a great quote that was posted on the entrance sign at my local gym.

*"If you don't
take care of your body,
where will you live?"*

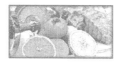

CHAPTER 6

Glycemic Index Chart

The glycemic index measures the increase in blood glucose (sugar) levels 2 to 3 hours after a meal. This measure does not factor in the amount of carbohydrates consumed. The "Glycemic load" factors in the amount of carbohydrates and provides a simpler way to determine which foods have less of an impact on your blood glucose levels.

Glycemic load is defined as grams of carbohydrates in the food multiplied by the GI index and then divided by 100. I know this sounds confusing but you don't really need to spend too much time understanding the calculations.

Here is a partial listing of foods provided by the American Diabetes Association.

Low GI Foods (55 or less)

- 100% stone-ground whole wheat or pumpernickel bread
- Oatmeal (rolled or steel-cut), oat bran, muesli
- Pasta, converted rice, barley, bulgar

- Sweet potato, corn, yam, lima/butter beans, peas, legumes and lentils
- Most fruits, non-starchy vegetables and carrots

Medium GI Foods (56-69)

- Whole wheat, rye and pita bread
- Quick oats
- Brown, wild or basmati rice, couscous

High GI Foods (70 or more)

- White bread or bagel
- Corn flakes, puffed rice, bran flakes, instant oatmeal
- Short grain white rice, rice pasta, macaroni and cheese from mix
- Russet potato, pumpkin
- Pretzels, rice cakes, popcorn, saltine crackers
- Melons and pineapples

When I first read through the list, I was a bit bummed that Pretzels and crackers were at the high end of the list. Pretzels were my late night go to food. You can find more detailed lists on the web, just search for Glycemic index chart or list and you will find numerous sites with listings.

The reason I included this section is to make you aware of how your body processes different types of food. High GI foods spike your blood sugar levels which usually creates a sugar high followed by a crash a few hours later. Since your body is unable to use all of the sugar that is produced, it has no choice but to turn those calories into fat. The exception to this is when it comes to endurance athletes. Their bodies are burning substantially more calories during long workouts and can convert the sugars immediately to energy. Even when they are not working out, they have conditioned their muscles to store higher levels of glycogen. This means they can consume more carbohydrates and convert them to glycogen instead of fat to be used during their next workout.

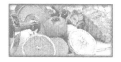

CHAPTER 7

Carb Cycle Diet Plan

Have you read chapter 2? If not go back and read it before you start. The first time I attempted this diet I didn't have the right foods in the house. I started with a low-carb day, by 3pm I had consumed 55% of my calories from carbs and I was still starving. I ended up at a local BBQ place eating a pulled pork sandwich with a pint of beer. Obviously a restart was going to be required. I spent the next day at my local warehouse club searching for good sources of protein, carbohydrates and fats.

My suggestion would be to take the first week and just monitor your current food intake using the MyFitnessPal application. If you are like me you will find that upwards of 80% of your calories are coming from carbohydrates. I would have cereal for breakfast, a bagel or waffles as a snack, a sandwich for lunch and then Pasta and some type of protein for dinner. I think it is important for you to understand where you are today before you attempt to make the change.

Remember it is OK to fail, as long as you dust yourself off and get back on the horse. The first couple of low carbohydrate days may be tough. If you have to start with one low carbohydrate day and two regular carbohydrate days for the first week, that is OK and certainly better than giving up.

Here is the plan

1. Setup an account on MyFitnesspal.com and determine how many calories you should eat per day.

2. Calculate the grams of protein, carbohydrates and fat you need on low-carb and high-carb days.

3. Review the shopping list and recipes, plan out your meals for the first week. I realize this will take some time but it is a worth while exercise, no pun intended.

4. Hit the store and purchase what you need for the first week

5. Decide on a workout plan and schedule your workouts for your high carb days.

6. Keep track of your diet, exercise and results using the journal at the back of the book or the printable journal available at the website.

7. Cycle!!

Sample Menu for a Low Carb Day

Goal: 20% carbs / 50% protein / 30% fat

- **Breakfast: Egg/Vegetable Omelet (LC)**
  Calories:305 / Carbs:4g / Protein:33g / Fat:16g

- **Snack: Yogurt with Fresh Fruit (HC)**
  Calories:160 / Carbs:27g / Protein:14g / Fat:0g

- **Lunch: Sausage & Chicken Salad with Green Beans (LC)**
  Calories:464 / Carbs:8g / Protein:47g / Fat:28g

- **Snack: Low Carb Protein Shake (LC)**
  Calories:270 / Carbs:9g / Protein:16g / Fat:20g

- **Dinner: Roast Pork & Broccoli (LC)**
  Calories:300 / Carbs:12g / Protein:48g / Fat:6g

- **Snack: Unsalted Mixed Nuts (LC)**
  Calories:190 / Carbs:7g / Protein:5g / Fat:16g

All of this food adds up to just 1,689 calories. If you include any high carb meals in your low carb day, just make sure to eat them earlier in the day. This menu breaks down to 21% carbs, 52% protein and 27% fat. If you need to increase calories you can double the protein portions on some of the dishes.

Sample Menu for a High Carb Day
Goal: 45% carbs / 40% protein / 15% fat

- **Breakfast: Egg Sandwich**
  Calories:270 / Carbs:22g / Protein:18g / Fat: 12g

- **Snack: Banana Protein Shake & 2 Kashi 7 Grain Waffles**
  Calories:453 / Carbs:47g / Protein:21g / Fat:11g

- **Lunch: FlatBread Grilled Chicken Wrap**
  Calories:371 / Carbs:23 g/ Protein:37 g/ Fat:18.6 **g**

- **Snack: Fage 2% Fat Blueberry Greek Yogurt**
  Calories:120 / Carbs:17g / Protein:13 g/ Fat:0g

- **Dinner: Broiled Fish Fillet**
  Calories:286 / Carbs:4 g/ Protein:19 g/ Fat:23g

  1/2 Cup Long Grain Brown Rice
   Calories:108 / Carbs:22g/ Protein:2g / Fat:1g

  1 Cup Steamed Broccoli
   Calories:54 / Carbs:12 g/ Protein:4 g/ Fat:0g

- **Snack: Fage Fat Free flavored Yogurt**
  Calories:120 / Carbs:17g / Protein:13 g/ Fat:0 g

The high carb sample menu comes in at 1,782 calories, the nutrients break down to 46% carbs, 36% protein and 18% fats, pretty close to the baseline. If your daily carbs are lower or higher, you can adjust portions or remove items to get to the correct level.

You don't have to hit the percentages exactly or the calories for that matter. As long as you are getting close each day you are fine, within 5% and say 200 calories. If carbohydrates make up a fair amount of your diet today, it will take you some time to make the transition. Stick with the diet for at least 30 days and you should see signs that it is working to reduce weight and fat and increase your energy and health.

One thing you will notice with the sample menus above is that you will be eating a fair amount of food throughout the day. The reason you can do this is because you are removing all of the bad foods from your diet. Soda, chips, candy, pretzels, all those foods you used to grab for a quick snack.

Here are a few sites with recipes and menu choices for carb cycling. If you search the web for Carb Cycling Diets and Carb Cycling recipes, you will find many more options to choose from.

http://www.scrawnytobrawny.com/fat-burning-machine

http://www.fitnesslynn.com/mealpln2.htm

http://www.livestrong.com/article/331452-menus-for-the-carb-cycling-diet/

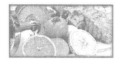

CHAPTER 8

Carb Cycling Recipes

Carb Cycling Recipes

The recipes are broken down into three sections; breakfast, lunch and dinner, and snacks. Each recipe is coded as HC (High Carb) or LC (Low Carb). I tried to provide a sampling of simple dishes you can incorporate into your diet. You can add in as many of your own recipes just follow the macro-nutrient percentages to align with your low and high carb days. The nutrition information next to each recipe is based on the ingredients I used, those numbers may vary based on the ingredients you have available. Your best bet is to enter the information into a calorie counting application to get accurate nutrition details for each of your meals.

You will find that many of the recipes use simple ingredients that you can prepare in advance. That is the key to your success, especially for your lunch and snacks. If you work in an office, then your meals need to be prepped and ready to go with just the help of a microwave. A number of the ingredients come directly from my local warehouse club. Some are pre-cooked which saves you time and effort but usually at the expense of higher sodium levels. The healthiest option is to prepare and cook your base ingredients in advance and have them ready to add to your meals. If time doesn't permit that, then the pre-cooked options can fill the gap.

You want to make this as simple as possible for yourself. Especially for breakfast and lunch, most people take the time to prepare dinner but rush through breakfast and lunch. You want to eat your larger meals earlier in the day not at the end of the day. Think about your diet today, perhaps you have a quick breakfast of cereal or a bagel, couple of snacks, a frozen processed meal for lunch and then by dinner time you are starving. You break out the pasta, bread or other carbohydrates to fill the void. Dinner is over, you hit the couch to watch some TV and then head off to bed to allow all those carbohydrates to convert into fat.

My intent is to continue to expand the recipe section of this book. If you have a recipe you would like to share, you can email them to me Jesse.Morgan@controlyourday.net. Please include the ingredients list, the recipe and a photo of the dish and let me know if you would like me to credit you for the recipe in the book.

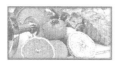

CHAPTER 9

Breakfast Recipes

Egg/Vegetable Omelet (LC)
Calories:305 / Carbs:4g / Protein:33g / Fat:16g

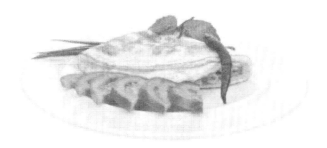

- 2 whole organic eggs
- 2/3 cup egg whites
- 1 ounce shredded part-skim mozzarella cheese
- 1/2 cup of tomatoes, diced

- Canola Oil cooking spray
- Omelet pan (7 to 10" pan)

Beat the eggs and egg whites in a small bowl and dice up the tomato if you want to include it in the omelet or you can just dress the plate with the them. Lightly spray the pan with cooking spray and then heat. Add the tomatoes and cook them for 3 to 5 minutes, moving them around the pan. Remove the tomatoes and add the egg mixture. Cook the egg mixture over medium heat until it is firm not runny. Add the tomatoes and cheese to one side of the omelet and then fold the omelet over and cook for another 2 to 3 minutes.

Greek Omelet (LC)

Calories:223 / Carbs:7g / Protein:20g / Fat:13g / Sugar:4g / Sodium:523mg

- 1 cup fresh spinach washed, dried and chopped
- 2 tbsp chopped roasted red pepper
- 1 egg white
- 2 whole eggs
- 2 tbsp feta cheese
- 5 cherry tomatoes, halved
- 1/2 tsp black pepper

Heat a small non-stick pan over medium low heat. Add spinach and roasted red pepper and cook for one minute, strain any excess liquid. Scramble egg whites and pour over spinach. Cover pan and cook for five minutes until eggs are fully cooked. Sprinkle over feta cheese and cherry tomatoes, fold omelet in half, transfer to your plate and sprinkle with pepper.

Western Omelet (LC)

Calories:246 / Carbs:8g / Protein:20g / Fat:13g / Sugar:5g / Sodium:647mg

- 2 tbsp onion, chopped
- 1/2 cup red or green pepper, chopped
- 1/4 cup mushrooms, chopped
- 3 slices deli ham, chopped
- 3 egg whites
- 1/2 tsp pepper
- 2 tbsp Colby jack cheese

Heat a small pan over medium heat. Spray with nonstick spray and add onions, peppers, and mushrooms. Cook until tender, about 3 minutes. Meanwhile mix egg whites and black pepper in a small bowl. Once veggies are cooked, reduce heat to medium-low, add ham and pour over eggs. Cover, and let cook for 5 minutes. Remove cover, sprinkle over cheese, fold in half and enjoy!

The Best Scrambled Eggs (LC)

Calories:169 / Carbs:9g / Protein:21g / Fat:5g / Sugar:6g / Sodium:477mg

- 2 large egg whites
- 1 large egg
- 1/4 cup fat free cottage cheese
- 8 cherry tomatoes, sliced in half
- 1/2 tsp pepper

Heat a small nonstick skillet over medium heat. Add egg whites, whole egg, and cottage cheese to a bowl and whisk. Stir in tomatoes and pepper and cook for 5 minutes.

Egg Sandwich (HC)

Calories:270 / Carbs:22g / Protein:18g / Fat:12g

- 1 whole organic egg

- 100 calorie whole wheat/whole grain sandwich thin

- 1 ounce shredded part-skim mozzarella cheese

- Canola Oil cooking spray

- 1 slice of tomato

Lightly spray the pan with cooking spray and then heat. Add the egg and break the yolk. Cook for 2 to 3 minutes and then flip the egg and add the cheese on top, 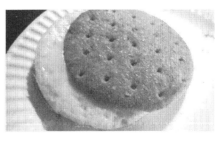 allow the cheese to melt. Place the tomato slice on the sandwich. I highly suggest picking up a single egg frying pan.

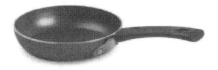

Open Faced Capri Egg Sandwiches (HC)

Calories:233 / Carbs:23g / Protein:20.5g / Fat:6.5g / Sugar:4.5 / Sodium:458mg

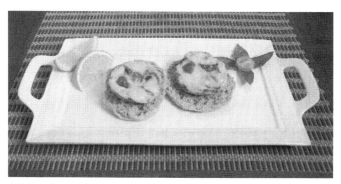

Makes 2 servings

- 4 egg whites
- 2 whole eggs
- 2 tbsp fat free milk
- 2 tbsp chopped scallions
- 8 cherry tomatoes sliced in half
- 2 tbsp low-fat mozzarella cheese
- 2 low-calorie, low carb English Muffins (Thomas 100 calorie multigrain)

Spray 4 slots of a muffin pan with nonstick spray. In a large bowl, beat eggs with milk until well combined. Stir in scallions, cherry tomatoes, and cheese. Pour the egg mixture into the muffin tins, dividing evenly into the four slots. Place eggs in oven and bake until done, about 20 minutes. Slice English muffins in half and serve each egg on a muffin half.

Steel Cut Oatmeal (HC)

Calories:330 / Carbs:38 g / Protein:31g / Fat: 6g /
Sugar:7g / Sodium:290mg

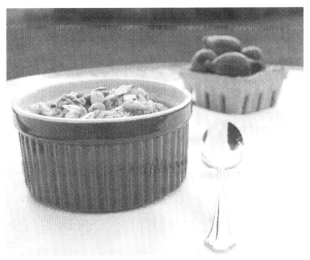

- 1 cup fat free milk
- 1/3 cup steel cut oats
- 1 tsp vanilla extract
- 1 tsp cinnamon
- 2 egg whites
- 1/2 cup fat free vanilla Greek yogurt
- 1 tbsp slivered almonds

Heat milk in a small saucepan until almost boiling. Reduce heat to low, stir in oats, vanilla extract, and cinnamon and cover. Cook for 15 minutes, stirring occasionally. Once cooked, remove cover, stir in egg whites, and cook for 1 additional minute.

Remove from heat and pour into bowl. Top with Greek yogurt, and almonds.

Egg/Vegetable Omelet (LC)
Calories:305 / Carbs:4g / Protein:33g / Fat:16g

- 2 whole organic eggs
- 2/3 cup egg whites
- 1 ounce shredded part-skim mozzarella cheese
- 1/2 cup of Tomatoes
- Canola Oil cooking spray
- Omelet pan (7 to 10" pan)

Beat the eggs and egg whites in a small bowl and dice up the tomato if you want to include it in the omelet or you can just dress the plate with the them. Lightly spray the pan with cooking spray and then heat. Add the tomatoes and cook them for 3 to 5 minutes, moving them around the pan. Remove the tomatoes and add the egg mixture. Cook the egg mixture over medium heat until it is firm not runny. Add the tomatoes and cheese to one side of the omelet and then fold the omelet over and cook for another 2 to 3 minutes.

Low Carb Protein Shake (LC)
Calories:270 / Carbs:9g / Protein:16g / Fat:20g

- 1/3 Cup CytoSport Muscle Milk Powder (or similar whey protein)
- 1 cup shredded ice

- 1 cup water
- 1 tablespoon flaxseed oil

Blend the ingredients together and enjoy. If you need to increase calories or protein for the day, add a second scoop and some additional water to the mix.

Blueberry Protein Shake (HC)
Calories:300 / Carbs:18g / Protein:16g / Fat:20g

- 1/3 Cup CytoSport Muscle Milk Powder (or similar whey protein)
- 1 cup shredded ice
- 1 cup water
- 1 tablespoon flaxseed oil
- 1/2 cup frozen blueberries

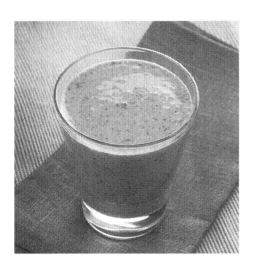

You should pickup a small portable blender to make the shakes. Cleanup is a breeze and you can even make them at work.

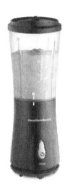

Blueberry Breakfast Smoothie (HC)

Calories:348 / Carbs:33 g / Protein:33 g / Fat:9 g / Sugar:26 g / Sodium:592mg

- 1/2 cup fat free vanilla Greek yogurt
- 1/2 cup low fat cottage cheese
- 1/2 cup fresh or frozen blueberries
- 1/2 cup ice
- 1 cup 2% milk

Blend all ingredients until smooth and enjoy.

Banana Protein Shake (HC)

Calories:203 / Carbs:23g / Protein:17g / Fat:6g

- 1/3 Cup CytoSport Muscle Milk Powder (or similar whey protein)
- 1 cup shredded ice
- 1 cup water
- 1/2 banana

Caffeinated Power Shake (LC)

Calories:373 / Carbs:12g / Protein:18g / Fat:30g

- 1/3 Cup CytoSport Muscle Milk Powder (or similar whey protein)
- 1 cup shredded ice
- 1/2 cup coconut milk
- 1 cup coffee (cold)
- 1 tablespoon flaxseed oil

This one has it all covered, protein, fat and a caffeine boost to fire up your day. Your workmates may never look at you the same way again.

Cocoa Coffee Breakfast Smoothie (HC)

Calories:237 / Carbs:22 / Protein:20 / Fat:9 / Sugar:18 / Sodium:158

- 1 cup brewed coffee, cold
- 1 1/2 tbsp cocoa powder
- 1 cup whole milk
- 1/2 cup fat free vanilla Greek yogurt
- 1 cup ice

Add all ingredients to blender and blend until smooth, about 30 seconds.

Yogurt with Fresh fruit (HC)

Calories:160 / Carbs:27g / Protein:14g / Fat:0g

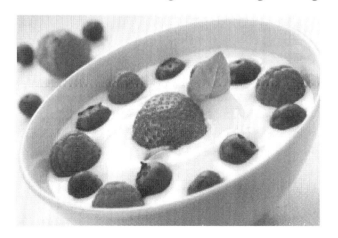

- 1 cup Chobani Vanilla Non-Fat Greek Yogurt
- 1/2 cup blueberries, raspberries or strawberries

You can switch out the brand and flavor of yogurt. If you go with fruit flavored yogurts, watch the amount of sugar.

Plain Yogurt (LC)

Calories:170/ Carbs:9 / Protein:23g / Fat:5g

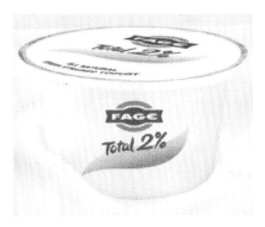

Greek yogurt makes a great snack, it has a higher percentage of protein then regular yogurt. I will admit the plain is not very tasty. You can drizzle in some honey or maple syrup to give it some flavor. You can buy the flavored version, but that will increase the percentage of carbohydrates and sugar. FAGE is my favorite, there are many to choose from, find the one that tastes best to you.

Fruit and Yogurt Parfait (HC)

Calories:360 / Carbs:40g / Protein:34g / Fat:10g / Sugar:23g / Sodium 347.5mg

- 1 cup fat free vanilla Greek yogurt
- 1/4 cup cottage cheese
- 1/4 cup sliced strawberries
- 1/4 cup blueberries
- 1/4 cup high protein granola (such as Bear Naked)

In a small bowl, mix Greek yogurt with cottage cheese until well blended. Take a tall glass and lay a third of the yogurt mixture on the bottom. Top with a portion of strawberries, blueberries and granola. Continue to layer until all ingredients are used.

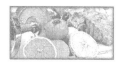

CHAPTER 10

Lunch-Dinner Recipes

Lunch-Dinner

Citrus Chicken Salad (HC)

Calories:299 / Carbs:16g / Protein:29g / Fat:16g / Sugar:13g / Sodium:84

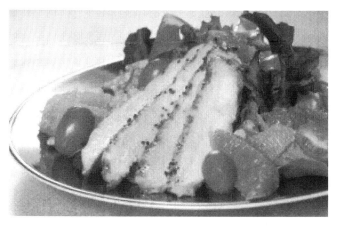

- 3 ounces of cooked chicken

- 1 cup of mixed greens

- 1 cup of red grapefruit

- 1 tablespoon olive oil

  Dash of red wine vinegar

- Handful of cherry or grape tomatoes

If you shop at Costco, you can put this entire meal together in 5 minutes. They sell pre-cooked chicken strips and single serve cups of red grapefruit, all you need to do is slice up the tomatoes, wash the mixed greens and your meal is ready to go. If you use the pre-cooked chicken, you will need to add 330mg of sodium to the nutrition information for this recipe, that is the downside to buying food pre-cooked. If you prefer to make everything fresh, then I suggest you cook your chicken breasts on Sunday so you have them for the week. If you need more calories/protein, you can double the serving size for the chicken.

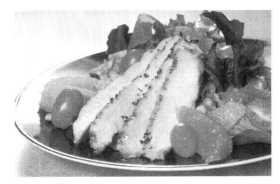

The carbs in this dish come from the grapefruit. If you leave the grapefruit out, you will end up with only 3 grams of carbohydrates and 2 grams of sugar.

Sausage & Chicken Salad with Green Beans (LC)
Calories:464 / Carbs:8g / Protein:47g / Fat:28g / Sugar:4g / Sodium:817mg

- 3 ounces of cooked chicken
- 1 pre-cooked chicken sausage link
- 1 cup of mixed greens
- 1 cup of string beans
- 1 tablespoon olive oil
- Dash of red wine vinegar
- 1 ounce of low-fat part-skim mozzarella shredded cheese

Steam frozen or fresh string beans. You can steam extra and put them in the refrigerator for use with other recipes. Boil, grill or microwave the chicken sausage, it is pre-cooked so you just need to heat it up. If you use the microwave, I suggest putting it in a glass bowl with small amount of water, that way it won't dry out. You can heat the grilled chicken in the microwave for 40 seconds or serve it chilled.

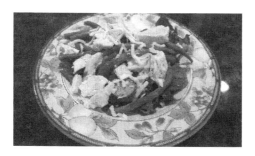

Place a bed of mix greens in the bowl, slice up and add the sausage, chicken and green beans. Drizzle the olive oil and red wine vinegar over the salad and then add the mozzarella cheese. A pinch of salt and pepper completes this simple dish.

Chicken & Avocado Salad (LC)

Calories:388 / Curbs.9g / Protein:20g / Fat:38g / Sugar:3g / Sodium:77mg

- 3 ounces of cooked chicken
- 1 cup of mixed greens
- 1/2 avocado
- 1 tablespoon olive oil
- Dash of red wine vinegar
- 1/2 sliced Roma Tomato

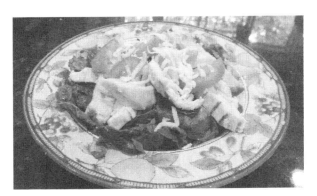

Another simple meal as long as you have the chicken prepared in advance. You can heat the chicken before you place it on the salad or just serve it cold. If your normal lunch is one of those frozen processed box lunches, this is a much healthier alternative.

Chicken Cesar Salad (LC)

Calories:290 / Carbs:15g / Protein:35g / Fat:10g / Sugar:2g / Sodium:436mg

- 1 head romaine lettuce, washed, dried and chopped
- 1 tbsp low-fat Cesar dressing
- 1 tbsp shredded parmesan cheese
- 4 oz boneless, skinless chicken breast, grilled
- 1/2 cup croutons

Add lettuce and Cesar dressing to a mixing bowl and toss until well coated. Transfer to a plate and top with cheese, chicken, and croutons.

Chicken Cobb Salad (LC)

Calories:431 / Carbs:20g / Protein:49g / Fat:15g / Sugar:8g / Sodium:677mg

- 3 cups romaine lettuce, washed, dried and chopped
- 1/2 cup cucumber, chopped
- 10 cherry tomatoes, halved
- 4 oz grilled chicken breast, chopped
- 1 boiled egg, chopped
- 2 strips microwave bacon, crumbled

- 1 oz low fat cheddar cheese
- 2 tbsp fat free ranch dressing

Lay lettuce down into a plate and top with cucumber, tomatoes, egg, bacon, and cheese. Drizzle ranch dressing over top and enjoy!

Cranberry & Chicken Spinach Salad (LC)

Calories:350 / Carbs:14g / Protein:37g / Fat:17g / Sugar:2.6g / Sodium:279.4mg

- 1 boneless skinless chicken breast, grilled
- 2 cups fresh baby spinach, washed and dried
- 1 tbsp walnuts, chopped
- 1 tbsp dried cranberries
- 2 tbsp feta cheese

Take grilled chicken breast and cut into small cubes. Place spinach on your plate and top with all remaining ingredients. Drizzle over fat-free dressing of choice.

Cranberry & Chicken Spinach Salad (LC)

Calories:350 / Carbs:14g / Protein:37g / Fat:17g / Sugar:2.6g / Sodium:279.4mg

- 1 boneless skinless chicken breast, grilled
- 2 cups fresh baby spinach, washed and dried
- 1 tbsp walnuts, chopped

- 1 tbsp dried cranberries
- 2 tbsp feta cheese

Take grilled chicken breast and cut into small cubes. Place spinach on your plate and top with all remaining ingredients. Drizzle over fat-free dressing of choice.

Chicken & Quinoa (HC)

Calories:429 / Carbs:44g / Protein:43g / Fat:8g / Sugar:3g / Sodium:745mg

- 1 cup cooked quinoa
- 4 oz boneless, skinless chicken breast, grilled
- 1/4 cup cucumber, sliced
- 1/4 cup low fat feta cheese
- 2 tbsp fat free Italian dressing

Add all ingredients to a bowl and stir to combine.

FlatBread Grilled Chicken Wrap (HC)

Calories:371 / Carbs:23g / Protein:37g / Fat:18.6g / Sugar:3g / Sodium:327mg

- 3 ounces of cooked chicken
- 1/2 cup mixed greens
- 1/2 cup diced tomatoes and red onion
- 1 tablespoon olive oil
- Dash of red wine vinegar

- 1 Flat out Flat bread or similar whole wheat tortilla

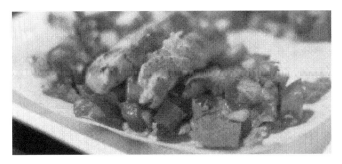

Very simple meal, all you have to do is put together the ingredients and enjoy. If you are at work, you might want to skip the red onion.

Fiesta Chicken Lettuce Cups (LC)

Calories:463 / Carbs:17g / Protein:41g / Fat:24g / Sugar:8g / Sodium:550mg

- 1 boneless skinless chicken breast, grilled
- 4-6 large leaves; iceberg or romaine lettuce
- 1/4 cup corn kernels
- 1/4 cup avocado, chopped
- 1/4 cup cilantro, chopped
- 2 tbsp scallions, chopped
- 2 tbsp salsa
- 2 tbsp sour cream
- 1/4 cup grated cheddar cheese

Cut grilled chicken breast into small cube pieces. Lay lettuce leaves down and distribute chicken, corn, avocado, cilantro and scallions evenly between the leaves. Top with salsa, sour cream, and cheese.

Chicken Soup (LC)

Calories:200 / Carbs:12g / Protein:25g / Fat:6g / Sugar:10g / Sodium:100mg

- Large organic chicken
- 1 cup chopped organic celery
- 1 lb organic carrots peeled and chopped 1/2 thick slices
- 1 bunch Italian parsley (rinsed and tied with cotton twine)
- 3 organic parsnips peeled and chopped 1/2 thick quarters
- 1 onion peeled, leave stem on end
- Better than Boullion organic chicken base

This is a family recipe that has been handed down from one generation to the next. This is not a quick recipe, it will take some time, but it is worth it. You can freeze what you don't eat to bring for lunch. I had to guess on the calories for this recipe, it will vary depending on the percentag you serve.

First of all, you should own a good chicken soup pot, I use a 12 quart stainless steel pot, which can be used to cook many other things. I do not believe in cooking in aluminum. Also have on hand cotton kitchen twine. Rinse the chicken off inside and out, cut off excess fat. Put in pot, cover with water, bring to a boil.

When it starts boiling, fat will rise to top of pot, keep skimming this white froth off, its a tedious job, but worth it. (You could also skin your chicken before boiling, but I find you lose some flavor), reducing the heat till it is simmering throughout the skimming process. I just use the pot top too hold the liquid I am skimming off and discarding in the sink. Add the carrots, parsley, parsnips and the celery at the very end.

Keep the pot simmering while adding all the above ingredients. Add the chicken base according to label directions. You will need to let this simmer about an hour or until the chicken is cooked. Usually I cook it until chicken starts to fall apart. The soup develops a better flavor the slower you simmer it. You do not want to overcook the vegetables, especially the celery as it will turn mushy. Keep the cover on the pot at a slight tilt.

After you shut the soup off and it cools somewhat, you can lift the chicken out carefully to a platter and de-bone it, discarding bones and skin, and cutting up the chicken meat, putting it back into the soup. Pull out the bunch of parsley and discard. You may also have to add salt to your taste. Sometimes as much as a tablespoon full. You can elect to have cooked white rice or brown rice or noodles in your bowl of chicken soup. Enjoy!

Chicken & Taco Soup (HC)

Calories:367 / Carbs:52g / Protein:44g / Fat:28g / Sugar:4.5g / Sodium:633mg

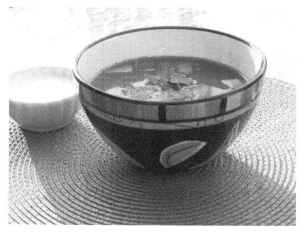

Makes 3 servings

- 1 lb boneless, skinless chicken breast
- 1/2 cup low sodium black beans
- 1 large zucchini, chopped
- 1/2 cup fresh or frozen corn kernels
- 1/2 cup green peppers, chopped
- 1/2 cup onion, chopped
- 1 cup canned, diced tomatoes
- 1 tbsp taco seasonings
- 1/2 tbsp chili powder
- 1/2 tbsp garlic powder
- 1 tsp crushed red pepper flakes

- 1/4 medium avocado, peeled and chopped
- 1/4 cup cilantro, chopped
- 1/4 cup fat free Greek yogurt

Add chicken and 8 cups of water to a large saucepan over high heat. Once water comes to a boil, reduce heat to low, cover, and cook until chicken is tender, about two hours. Add all remaining ingredients except for avocado, cilantro, and yogurt and continue cooking for ½ hour. Once cooked, serve soup, top with avocado, cilantro, and yogurt.

Turkey Burger Salad Plate (HC)

Calories:376 / Carbs:52g / Protein:44g / Fat:28g / Sugar:4.5g / Sodium:633mg

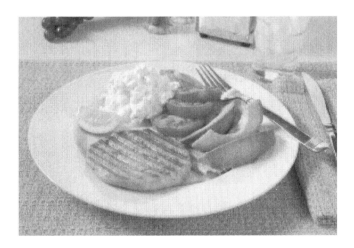

- 1 Turkey Burger
- 1/2 sliced avocado

- 1/4 cup cottage cheese

- 1/2 sliced Roma tomato

- 1 lemon wedge

Yes I know this does not look like the most exciting of meals, but it offers a great balance of fat, protein and carbs for a healthy high carb meal. Follow the instructions to cook your turkey burger, either on the grill, in a pan or a broiler.

There are a number of studies that show that adding lemon juice or vinegar to a meal can help to reduce the glycemic index rating by 20% or more.

The cottage cheese turns this meal from a low carb meal to a high carb meal. If you skip the cottage cheese, drop the calories by 40, the carbs by 40 and the sodium by 230 and you have a LC version of the same dish.

Turkey Lettuce Wraps (LC)

Calories:201 / Carbs:10.4g / Protein:21.5g / Fat:12.4g / Sugar:5.1g / Sodium:920mg

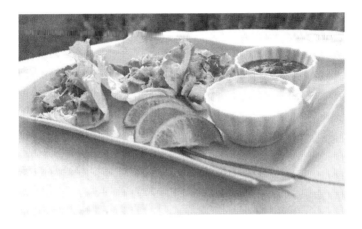

- 4 large lettuce leaves, iceberg or romaine works well
- 2 tbsp plain fat free Greek Yogurt
- 8 slices thinly sliced turkey breast
- 1/2 cucumber, quartered lengthwise
- 1/4 cup shredded cheddar cheese

Lay lettuce leaves down and distribute yogurt evenly on each leaf. Lay two slices of turkey, one slice of cucumber and 1 table-spoon of cheddar cheese on each leaf. Roll up each leaf and enjoy.

Spaghetti Squash with Turkey Meatballs (HC)

Calories:353 / Carbs:36g / Protein:31g / Fat:11g / Sugar:16g / Sodium:929mg

- 1 small spaghetti squash
- 1/2 cup fat free tomato sauce
- 1/4 cup fat free ricotta cheese
- 4 pre-cooked turkey meatballs
- 2 tbsp chopped basil
- 1/2 tsp each, salt and pepper
- 1 tsp crushed red pepper flakes

Poke a few holes around the spaghetti squash and cook in microwave until soft, about 8 minutes. Once cooked, slice in half and remove seeds. Using a fork, scrape out the spaghetti squash and transfer to a bowl. Add the tomato sauce and ricotta cheese and mix until well distributed. Top your squash with heated meatballs (follow instructions on package), basil, salt, pepper and red pepper flakes.

Turkey Stuffed Peppers (HC)

Calories:484 / Carbs:48g / Protein:36g / Fat:17g / Sugar:10g / Sodium:447mg

- 1 tbsp olive oil
- 4 oz lean ground turkey
- 1/4 cup canned kidney beans, strained
- 1/2 cup diced tomatoes
- 1/2 cup cooked brown rice

- 1 tsp chili powder
- 1 tsp garlic powder
- 1/2 tsp pepper
- 2 whole green peppers, washed

Place a pan over medium heat and add olive oil. Once oil is hot, add ground turkey and cook until thoroughly cooked, about 8 minutes. Then, turn off heat and stir together all ingredients except for green peppers. Cut tops off the green peppers and fill each pepper with turkey mixture. Place peppers onto a baking dish, add an inch of water and cover with tinfoil. Bake at 350 for 35 minutes, remove from oven and let sit for 5 to 10 minutes.

Grilled Pork Loin & Broccoli (LC)

Calories:300/ Carbs:12g / Protein:48g / Fat:6g / Sugar:2g / Sodium:160mg

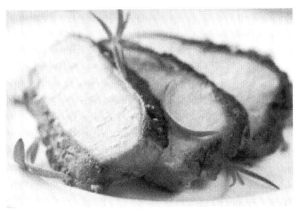

- 2 pork loins (6 oz serving size)
- 2 heads of broccoli (1 cup serving size)

- 2 oranges & 1 lime

- 5 cloves of garlic

This recipe comes direct from good friend of mine in New Jersey that loves to cook. I have never had a bad meal with the man.

For the Pork, buy TENDERLOINS, which typically come in 2 loins to a pack. They are in the glorious pork section of the supermarket usually above the picnic hams and pork loins. Make sure they are tenderloins. A package of 2 should feed 4. For the marinade, squeeze the juice of 2 oranges and 1 lime (no lemon!) into a zip lock baggie. Crush 4-5 cloves of garlic (don't be shy, it's heaven) and dump it into the bag. Wash the tenderloins and pat dry with a paper towel. Don't eat the paper towel. Salt and pepper the tenderloins to taste. Don't be afraid of the salt, pork loves salt and it won't be salty. A good palmful will do nicely. Put the tenderloins in the bag, push out the air, give a little shake and shimmy, place in the fridge for 1-4 hours. Put it on a plate in the bag in the fridge to catch any drippings. Too easy.

The broccoli is easy – 2 heads of broccoli, removing the stems so you have nice florets. Don't cut them too shy, most of the nutrients are closer to the stem so showing a little stem is good, plus, it presents better. Wash the broccoli and place in a microwave safe bowl. Don't shake the broccoli too much after washing as the trapped water will help it cook. The bowl should have a little bit of water in it so it can steam. To cook, place the bowl in the microwave with a

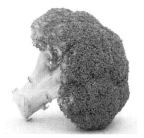

paper towel over it to trap the steam. 3 minutes should do it. I like the broccoli a bit firm and no mush. When it's done, dump the water, transfer to a serving dish, salt, pepper and a little butter and your in heaven.

Here is the time line to prepare this perfect meal ready at 7pm

- 1:00pm: Pork in marinade in the fridge

- 5:30pm: Take pork out of the fridge

- 6:00pm: Fire up the grill

- 6:30pm: Place pork on grill, use PAM on grill or rub olive oil on grill with paper towel. Keep grill between 400 and 425. Turn the pork a couple times to brown, but don't open the grill too often. Cook to an internal temperature of 145 degrees as recommended by the USDA.

- 6:52pm: Take pork off grill

- 6:55pm: Start broccoli in the microwave

- 7:00pm: High 5 the family, toast to a successful operation and enjoy your meal!

Quick Mix Meatloaf (LC)

Calories:245 / Carbs:9.3g / Protein:19g / Fat:12g / Sugar:2.5g / Sodium:160mg

Makes 6 servings

- 1 lb 93% lean ground beef (grass fed if possible)
- 2 large eggs
- 2 tbsp ketchup
- 1/2 cup carrots, shredded
- 1/4 cup onion, shredded
- 3/4 cup dry oats, traditional or quick cooking
- 1 tsp garlic powder
- 1 tsp pepper
- 2 tbsp olive oil
- Preheat oven to 350 degrees.

In a large bowl combine all ingredients, except for olive oil, and mix until well incorporated. Transfer meatloaf onto a large baking sheet and form into a log, about 8 inches long. Drizzle olive oil over meatloaf and bake for 45 minutes or until temperature reaches 160 degrees. Remove from oven, let rest on counter for 5-10 minutes.

Steak, Peppers and Onions (HC)

Calories:496 / Carbs:57g / Protein:47g / Fat:10g / Sugar:5g / Sodium:723mg

- 4 oz lean shaved steak
- 1/2 cup green pepper, sliced

- 1/2 cup onions, sliced
- 2 slices fat free provolone cheese
- 1 cup cooked brown rice

Heat a nonstick pan over medium heat. Add steak, peppers, and onions and cook for ten minutes stirring often. Add cheese and allow to melt. Place cooked brown rice onto your plate and top with steak.

Broiled Fish Fillet (LC)

Calories:286 / Carbs:4g / Protein:19g / Fat:23g / Sugar:2g / Sodium:621mg

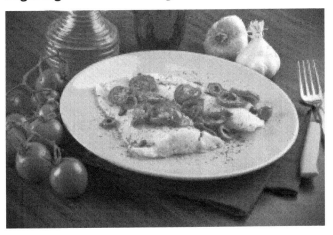

- 1 white fish fillet
- 1/2 cup sliced cherry tomatoes
- 1/4 cup green olives sliced
- 1 tablespoon olive oil
- 3 cloves of garlic

- Salt & Pepper
- A few basil leaves torn into pieces

This is a great single serve or family meal, just increase the portions for each ingredient as needed.

Preheat oven to 425 degrees Fahrenheit. Combine the tomatoes, olives, oil, garlic and basil in a 9 by 13 inch baking pan, add salt and pepper as needed. Roast for 15 minutes and then add the fish fillets on top of the mixture. Roast for 10 minutes or until fish is no longer translucent. Place fish on a serving dish and spoon out the tomato and olive mixture across the top of the fish.

Shrimp with Cheddar Grits (HC)

Calories:433 / Carbs:38g / Protein:34g / Fat:13g / Sugar:2g / Sodium:584mg

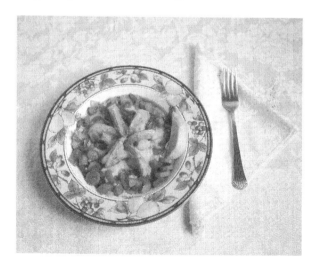

- 1/4 cup dry quick cooking grits

- 1/4 cup chopped green pepper
- 2 tbsp chopped onion
- 1 clove minced garlic
- 1/4 cup chopped celery
- 4 ounces light beer
- 8 jumbo shrimp peeled and de-veined
- 1/2 tsp black pepper
- 1/4 cup cheddar cheese
- 1 lemon wedge

Pour grits into small saucepan and cook according to package directions. Meanwhile, place a pan over medium heat and spray with nonstick spray. Add green pepper, onion, garlic and celery, cook for five minutes. Once green pepper is tender, add beer and shrimp to pan; cover and cook for an additional five minutes. Remove from heat and add pepper. Once grits are cooked, remove from heat and stir in cheddar cheese until well combined. Place grits on bottom of your plate and top with shrimp and vegetable mixture. Serve with a wedge of lemon.

Pesto Prosciutto Shrimp with Green Beans (HC)

Calories:291 / Carbs:9g / Protein:29g / Fat:16g / Sugar:2g / Sodium:1141mg

- 6 jumbo shrimp, peeled and deveined
- 2 cloves garlic, minced
- 6 large basil leaves
- 3 slices, thinly sliced prosciutto, sliced in half

- 1 cup raw green beans, washed

Place shrimp in a small bowl and coat with garlic. Take each piece of shrimp and wrap one basil leaf and one piece of prosciutto around. Use a skewer to secure the basil and prosciutto on each shrimp. Cook shrimp on a grill over medium heat for 3 minutes on each side. Meanwhile, place green beans in a bowl with an inch of water, cover with plastic wrap and microwave for three minutes. Serve shrimp with green beans on the side.

Zucchini Noodle Lasagna (HC)
Calories:233 / Carbs:25.5g / Protein:21g / Fat:7g / Sugar:13.5g / Sodium:993.5mg

Makes 2 servings

- 1/2 cup fat free mozzarella cheese
- 3/4 cup low fat ricotta cheese
- 1 tsp garlic powder
- 1/2 tsp each of salt and pepper
- 2 medium zucchini, sliced thin lengthwise
- 1/2 cup green pepper, sliced
- 1 cup baby bella mushrooms, thinly sliced

1 cup fat free pizza sauce Preheat oven to 375 degrees. In a small bowl, mix together mozzarella cheese, ricotta cheese, garlic powder, salt, and pepper until well combined. Spray a 9x9 inch pan with nonstick spray. Place thin strips of zucchini on the bottom of the pan until bottom is covered. Sprinkle on some green pepper and mushrooms and top with 1/3 C sauce and 1/3 of ricotta mixture. Top with more zucchini strips and continue

layering until all ingredients are used. Place pan into preheated oven and cook for 30 minutes. Remove from oven, allow to cool for a few minutes.

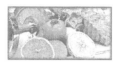

CHAPTER 11

Snacks

Summer Veggie & Herb Cottage Cheese (LC)

Calories:343 / Carbs:12g / Protein:32g / Fat:18g / Sugar:3g / Sodium:923mg

- 1 cup 2% fat cottage cheese
- 1 tbsp fresh basil, chopped
- 1 tbsp fresh parsley, chopped
- 1 tbsp fresh chives, chopped
- 1 tbsp fresh oregano, chopped
- 1 tsp pepper
- 5 cherry tomatoes, halved
- 1/4 cup cucumber, chopped
- 1 tbsp olive oil

In a bowl, mix together cottage cheese, basil, parsley, chives oregano, and pepper until well combined. Top with tomatoes, cucumber, olive oil.

Unsalted Mixed Nuts (LC)

Calories:200 / Carbs:7g / Protein:5g / Fat:17g / Sugar:1g / Sodium:120mg

Serving size is 1/4 cup or about 30 pieces. If you are going to use these as a snack, make sure to dole out your serving in advance, otherwise you could easily blow out your fat and calories for the day if you keep reaching in for more.

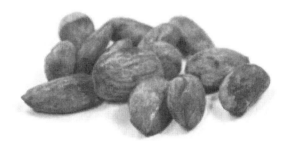

Hummus with Pita & Vegetables (HC)

Calories:261 / Carbs:28g / Protein:11g / Fat:12g / Sugar:8g / Sodium:678mg

- 1 cup organic celery
- 1 cup carrots
- 1 single serving cup of Sabra Classic Hummus
- 1 Joseph's Oat Bran & Whole Wheat Pita Bread

This is a simple snack, great for an afternoon pick me up. It does have a higher level of sodium from the hummus and the pita breads. You should be able to find low sodium alternatives to reduce the salt if that is a concern.

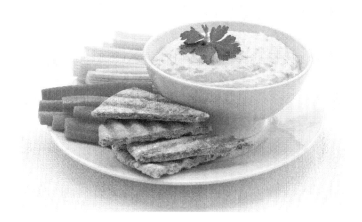

Mixed Greens with Avocado (LC)

Calories:244 / Carbs:7g / Protein:1.5g / Fat:35g / Sugar:1g / Sodium:10mg

- 1 cup mixed greens
- 1/2 avocado
- 1 teaspoon olive oil
- 2 teaspoons balsamic vinegar
- Fresh pepper
- Sliced small tomato
- 1/4 cucumber sliced

Slice the avocado on top of the mixed greens and then drizzle Olive oil and balsamic vinegar over the top. You can add a bit of protein to this snack to complete it.

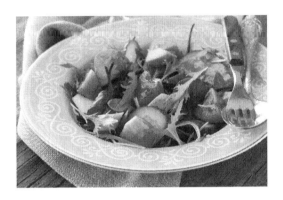

Mixed Greens with Egg (LC)

Calories:199 / Carbs:0g / Protein:6g / Fat:19g / Sugar:0g / Sodium:70mg

- 1 cup mixed greens
- 1 hard boiled egg
- 1 teaspoon olive oil
- 2 teaspoons balsamic vinegar
- Fresh pepper

Slice the egg on the top of the mixed greens and then drizzle olive oil and balsamic vinegar over the top.

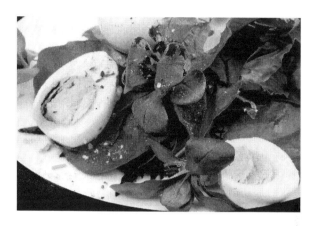

Egg Salad (LC)

Calories:218 / Carbs:10g / Protein:27g / Fat:7g / Sugar:4g / Sodium:847mg

- 2 boiled egg whites
- 1 whole boiled egg
- 1/2 cup fat free cottage cheese
- 2 tbsp low-fat mayonnaise
- 1/2 tsp pepper

Place eggs in bowl and break up with fork into small pieces. Stir in remaining ingredients until everything is well combined. Enjoy on a light English muffin for a high carb meal or over lettuce for a low carb meal.

Strawberries & Cream (HC)

Calories:174 / Carbs:19g / Protein:18g / Fat:19g / Sugar:15g / Sodium:272mg

- 1/2 cup 2% fat vanilla Greek yogurt
- 1/4 cup low fat cottage cheese
- 1 tsp vanilla extract
- 1 packet Stevia
- 1 cup strawberries, sliced

In a bowl, mix yogurt, cottage cheese, vanilla extract, and stevia until well combined. Stir in strawberries, transfer to a dessert dish.

Check out the breakfast recipes, many of them can double as snacks.

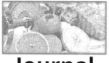

Journal

This journal was designed for use with the carb cycling diet. I think you will find that you can easily adapt it to a number of other diets as well.

Setup

1. Fill in your name, current weight and your goal weight. Your goal weight should be a bit of a stretch but still realistic. Set your initial goal weight for 6 weeks from the start of your diet. 1 to 2 pounds of weight loss a week would require burning 500 to 1,000 more calories than you consume each day.

2. Determine your daily caloric intake and enter it in the "Calories per day" box. You can get this information from a number of sites on the web.

3. Determine the allocations of macro-nutrients (proteins, carbs, fats) for low and high carb day and enter them on the next page. You will model your meals off this baseline information. See Chapter 3 for more information on how to define your levels.

Carb Cycling

1. If your week starts on Monday take a few minutes on Sunday afternoon and plan out your week. Check off the boxes that define the type of carb day and even give some thought to your workouts for the week. You can enter brief workout descriptions in to help with your planning.

2. On the first day of the week, record your weight

3. At the end of each day record your activity. You can chose to enter your macronutrients as servings, grams or percentage of calories.

4. Enter your total calories for the day, grams of sugar consumed, energy level and attitude. The last two can be any scale you want. For example you could use a scale of 1-5 or just put in words like high, cruddy, etc.

Wrapping up the week

1. At the end of each week log your weight (do it at the same time of day that you did at the beginning if the week.

2. Take a few moments to record your thoughts for the week.

SHOPPING LIST

Protein Sources

Eggs

Egg Whites

Skim Milk

Low fat Yogurt

Cottage Cheese - 1% Fat

Protein Powder

Tuna

Salmon

Shelfish

Chicken (skinless-white)

Lean Beef

Turkey (skinless-white)

Fruit Carbs

Apple

Apricot

Banana

Berry

Grape

Kiwi

Melon

Orange

Peach

Pear

Pineapple

Plum

Carbs

Beans/Legumes

Brown Rice

Corn

Oats

Peas

Popcorn

Potatoes

Quinoa

Sweet Potatos

Whole Grain Breads

Whole Grain Pasta

Wild Rice

Vegetables

Veggies

Peppers

Unions

Broccoli

Spinich

Green Beans

Asparagus

Carrots

Celery

Radishes

Cucumbers

Your Profile

Name	
Journal Start Date	
Starting Weight	
Goal Weight & Date	
Calories per day	

When you setup a profile on MyFitnessPal, it will recommend your daily caloric intake based on your activity level, age and weight.

High Carb Day	Servings	Grams	% of Calories
Carbohydrates			
Proteins			
Fats			

Low Carb Day	Servings	Grams	% of Calories
Carbohydrates			
Proteins			
Fats			

No Carb Day	Servings	Grams	% of Calories
Carbohydrates			
Proteins			
Fats			

*What is your goal? Dream it,
Define it Do it !*

Week # _____

Starting Weight: _____

Date/Day _____   **Carb Level:** ❏High ❏Low ❏No ❏Free

Nutrient	Servings	Grams	%
Carbs			
Protein			
Fat			

Total Calories	
Grams of Sugar	
Energy Level	
Attitude	

Workout:	Time:	Calories:

Date/Day _____   **Carb Level:** ❏High ❏Low ❏No ❏Free

Nutrient	Servings	Grams	%
Carbs			
Protein			
Fat			

Total Calories	
Grams of Sugar	
Energy Level	
Attitude	

Workout:	Time:	Calories:

Date/Day _____   **Carb Level:** ❏High ❏Low ❏No ❏Free

Nutrient	Servings	Grams	%
Carbs			
Protein			
Fat			

Total Calories	
Grams of Sugar	
Energy Level	
Attitude	

Workout:	Time:	Calories:

Date/Day _____   **Carb Level:** ❏High ❏Low ❏No ❏Free

Nutrient	Servings	Grams	%
Carbs			
Protein			
Fat			

Total Calories	
Grams of Sugar	
Energy Level	
Attitude	

Workout:	Time:	Calories:

Date/Day_____ **Carb Level:** ❏High ❏Low ❏No ❏Free

Nutrient	Servings	Grams	%
Carbs			
Protein			
Fat			

Total Calories	
Grams of Sugar	
Energy Level	
Attitude	

Workout:	Time:	Calories:

Date/Day_____ **Carb Level:** ❏High ❏Low ❏No ❏Free

Nutrient	Servings	Grams	%
Carbs			
Protein			
Fat			

Total Calories	
Grams of Sugar	
Energy Level	
Attitude	

Workout:	Time:	Calories:

Date/Day_____ **Carb Level:** ❏High ❏Low ❏No ❏Free

Nutrient	Servings	Grams	%
Carbs			
Protein			
Fat			

Total Calories	
Grams of Sugar	
Energy Level	
Attitude	

Workout:	Time:	Calories:

Ending Weight:

Notes

Drink more water!

Week # _____

Starting Weight: _____

Date/Day _____   **Carb Level:** ❏High   ❏Low   ❏No   ❏Free

Nutrient	Servings	Grams	%		
Carbs				Total Calories	
				Grams of Sugar	
Protein				Energy Level	
Fat				Attitude	

Workout:	Time:	Calories:

Date/Day _____   **Carb Level:** ❏High   ❏Low   ❏No   ❏Free

Nutrient	Servings	Grams	%		
Carbs				Total Calories	
				Grams of Sugar	
Protein				Energy Level	
Fat				Attitude	

Workout:	Time:	Calories:

Date/Day _____   **Carb Level:** ❏High   ❏Low   ❏No   ❏Free

Nutrient	Servings	Grams	%		
Carbs				Total Calories	
				Grams of Sugar	
Protein				Energy Level	
Fat				Attitude	

Workout:	Time:	Calories:

Date/Day _____   **Carb Level:** ❏High   ❏Low   ❏No   ❏Free

Nutrient	Servings	Grams	%		
Carbs				Total Calories	
				Grams of Sugar	
Protein				Energy Level	
Fat				Attitude	

Workout:	Time:	Calories:

Date/Day _____ Carb Level: ❑High ❑Low ❑No ❑Free

Nutrient	Servings	Grams	%
Carbs			
Protein			
Fat			

Total Calories	
Grams of Sugar	
Energy Level	
Attitude	

Workout:	Time:	Calories:

Date/Day _____ Carb Level: ❑High ❑Low ❑No ❑Free

Nutrient	Servings	Grams	%
Carbs			
Protein			
Fat			

Total Calories	
Grams of Sugar	
Energy Level	
Attitude	

Workout:	Time:	Calories:

Date/Day _____ Carb Level: ❑High ❑Low ❑No ❑Free

Nutrient	Servings	Grams	%
Carbs			
Protein			
Fat			

Total Calories	
Grams of Sugar	
Energy Level	
Attitude	

Workout:	Time:	Calories:

Ending Weight:

Notes

*Don't give up, the beginning is
always the hardest.*

Week # _____

Starting Weight: _____

Date/Day _____   **Carb Level:** ❏High ❏Low ❏No ❏Free

Nutrient	Servings	Grams	%
Carbs			
Protein			
Fat			

Total Calories	
Grams of Sugar	
Energy Level	
Attitude	

Workout:	Time:	Calories:

Date/Day _____   **Carb Level:** ❏High ❏Low ❏No ❏Free

Nutrient	Servings	Grams	%
Carbs			
Protein			
Fat			

Total Calories	
Grams of Sugar	
Energy Level	
Attitude	

Workout:	Time:	Calories:

Date/Day _____   **Carb Level:** ❏High ❏Low ❏No ❏Free

Nutrient	Servings	Grams	%
Carbs			
Protein			
Fat			

Total Calories	
Grams of Sugar	
Energy Level	
Attitude	

Workout:	Time:	Calories:

Date/Day _____   **Carb Level:** ❏High ❏Low ❏No ❏Free

Nutrient	Servings	Grams	%
Carbs			
Protein			
Fat			

Total Calories	
Grams of Sugar	
Energy Level	
Attitude	

Workout:	Time:	Calories:

Date/Day_____ **Carb Level:** ❑High ❑Low ❑No ❑Free

Nutrient	Servings	Grams	%
Carbs			
Protein			
Fat			

Total Calories	
Grams of Sugar	
Energy Level	
Attitude	

Workout:	Time:	Calories:

Date/Day_____ **Carb Level:** ❑High ❑Low ❑No ❑Free

Nutrient	Servings	Grams	%
Carbs			
Protein			
Fat			

Total Calories	
Grams of Sugar	
Energy Level	
Attitude	

Workout:	Time:	Calories:

Date/Day_____ **Carb Level:** ❑High ❑Low ❑No ❑Free

Nutrient	Servings	Grams	%
Carbs			
Protein			
Fat			

Total Calories	
Grams of Sugar	
Energy Level	
Attitude	

Workout:	Time:	Calories:

Ending Weight:

Notes

*A year from now, you will be happy
you stuck with this.*

Week # _____

Starting Weight: _____

Date/Day _____ **Carb Level:** ❑High ❑Low ❑No ❑Free

Nutrient	Servings	Grams	%
Carbs			
Protein			
Fat			

Total Calories	
Grams of Sugar	
Energy Level	
Attitude	

Workout:	Time:	Calories:

Date/Day _____ **Carb Level:** ❑High ❑Low ❑No ❑Free

Nutrient	Servings	Grams	%
Carbs			
Protein			
Fat			

Total Calories	
Grams of Sugar	
Energy Level	
Attitude	

Workout:	Time:	Calories:

Date/Day _____ **Carb Level:** ❑High ❑Low ❑No ❑Free

Nutrient	Servings	Grams	%
Carbs			
Protein			
Fat			

Total Calories	
Grams of Sugar	
Energy Level	
Attitude	

Workout:	Time:	Calories:

Date/Day _____ **Carb Level:** ❑High ❑Low ❑No ❑Free

Nutrient	Servings	Grams	%
Carbs			
Protein			
Fat			

Total Calories	
Grams of Sugar	
Energy Level	
Attitude	

Workout:	Time:	Calories:

Date/Day_____ **Carb Level:** ❑High ❑Low ❑No ❑Free

Nutrient	Servings	Grams	%
Carbs			
Protein			
Fat			

Total Calories	
Grams of Sugar	
Energy Level	
Attitude	

Workout:	Time:	Calories:

Date/Day_____ **Carb Level:** ❑High ❑Low ❑No ❑Free

Nutrient	Servings	Grams	%
Carbs			
Protein			
Fat			

Total Calories	
Grams of Sugar	
Energy Level	
Attitude	

Workout:	Time:	Calories:

Date/Day_____ **Carb Level:** ❑High ❑Low ❑No ❑Free

Nutrient	Servings	Grams	%
Carbs			
Protein			
Fat			

Total Calories	
Grams of Sugar	
Energy Level	
Attitude	

Workout:	Time:	Calories:

Ending Weight:

Notes

Each day brings you closer to your goal.

Week # _____

Starting Weight: _____

Date/Day _____ **Carb Level:** ❏High ❏Low ❏No ❏Free

Nutrient	Servings	Grams	%		
Carbs				Total Calories	
Protein				Grams of Sugar	
Fat				Energy Level	
				Attitude	

Workout:	Time:	Calories:

Date/Day _____ **Carb Level:** ❏High ❏Low ❏No ❏Free

Nutrient	Servings	Grams	%		
Carbs				Total Calories	
Protein				Grams of Sugar	
Fat				Energy Level	
				Attitude	

Workout:	Time:	Calories:

Date/Day _____ **Carb Level:** ❏High ❏Low ❏No ❏Free

Nutrient	Servings	Grams	%		
Carbs				Total Calories	
Protein				Grams of Sugar	
Fat				Energy Level	
				Attitude	

Workout:	Time:	Calories:

Date/Day _____ **Carb Level:** ❏High ❏Low ❏No ❏Free

Nutrient	Servings	Grams	%		
Carbs				Total Calories	
Protein				Grams of Sugar	
Fat				Energy Level	
				Attitude	

Workout:	Time:	Calories:

Date/Day _____ **Carb Level:** ❑High ❑Low ❑No ❑Free

Nutrient	Servings	Grams	%
Carbs			
Protein			
Fat			

Total Calories	
Grams of Sugar	
Energy Level	
Attitude	

Workout:	Time:	Calories:

Date/Day _____ **Carb Level:** ❑High ❑Low ❑No ❑Free

Nutrient	Servings	Grams	%
Carbs			
Protein			
Fat			

Total Calories	
Grams of Sugar	
Energy Level	
Attitude	

Workout:	Time:	Calories:

Date/Day _____ **Carb Level:** ❑High ❑Low ❑No ❑Free

Nutrient	Servings	Grams	%
Carbs			
Protein			
Fat			

Total Calories	
Grams of Sugar	
Energy Level	
Attitude	

Workout:	Time:	Calories:

Ending Weight:

Notes

Try to reduce the number of hours you spend sitting each day.

Week # _____

Starting Weight: _____

Date/Day _____ **Carb Level:** ❑High ❑Low ❑No ❑Free

Nutrient	Servings	Grams	%			
Carbs				Total Calories		
Protein				Grams of Sugar		
Fat				Energy Level		
				Attitude		

Workout:	Time:	Calories:

Date/Day _____ **Carb Level:** ❑High ❑Low ❑No ❑Free

Nutrient	Servings	Grams	%			
Carbs				Total Calories		
Protein				Grams of Sugar		
Fat				Energy Level		
				Attitude		

Workout:	Time:	Calories:

Date/Day _____ **Carb Level:** ❑High ❑Low ❑No ❑Free

Nutrient	Servings	Grams	%			
Carbs				Total Calories		
Protein				Grams of Sugar		
Fat				Energy Level		
				Attitude		

Workout:	Time:	Calories:

Date/Day _____ **Carb Level:** ❑High ❑Low ❑No ❑Free

Nutrient	Servings	Grams	%			
Carbs				Total Calories		
Protein				Grams of Sugar		
Fat				Energy Level		
				Attitude		

Workout:	Time:	Calories:

Date/Day _____ **Carb Level:** ❑High ❑Low ❑No ❑Free

Nutrient	Servings	Grams	%
Carbs			
Protein			
Fat			

Total Calories	
Grams of Sugar	
Energy Level	
Attitude	

Workout:	Time:	Calories:

Date/Day _____ **Carb Level:** ❑High ❑Low ❑No ❑Free

Nutrient	Servings	Grams	%
Carbs			
Protein			
Fat			

Total Calories	
Grams of Sugar	
Energy Level	
Attitude	

Workout:	Time:	Calories:

Date/Day _____ **Carb Level:** ❑High ❑Low ❑No ❑Free

Nutrient	Servings	Grams	%
Carbs			
Protein			
Fat			

Total Calories	
Grams of Sugar	
Energy Level	
Attitude	

Workout:	Time:	Calories:

Ending Weight:

Notes

Don't beat yourself up when you have a bad week, accept it and move forward.

Week # _____

Starting Weight: _____

Date/Day _____   **Carb Level:** ❑High ❑Low ❑No ❑Free

Nutrient	Servings	Grams	%
Carbs			
Protein			
Fat			

Total Calories	
Grams of Sugar	
Energy Level	
Attitude	

Workout:	Time:	Calories:

Date/Day _____   **Carb Level:** ❑High ❑Low ❑No ❑Free

Nutrient	Servings	Grams	%
Carbs			
Protein			
Fat			

Total Calories	
Grams of Sugar	
Energy Level	
Attitude	

Workout:	Time:	Calories:

Date/Day _____   **Carb Level:** ❑High ❑Low ❑No ❑Free

Nutrient	Servings	Grams	%
Carbs			
Protein			
Fat			

Total Calories	
Grams of Sugar	
Energy Level	
Attitude	

Workout:	Time:	Calories:

Date/Day _____   **Carb Level:** ❑High ❑Low ❑No ❑Free

Nutrient	Servings	Grams	%
Carbs			
Protein			
Fat			

Total Calories	
Grams of Sugar	
Energy Level	
Attitude	

Workout:	Time:	Calories:

Date/Day _____ **Carb Level:** ❏High ❏Low ❏No ❏Free

Nutrient	Servings	Grams	%
Carbs			
Protein			
Fat			

Total Calories	
Grams of Sugar	
Energy Level	
Attitude	

Workout:	Time:	Calories:

Date/Day _____ **Carb Level:** ❏High ❏Low ❏No ❏Free

Nutrient	Servings	Grams	%
Carbs			
Protein			
Fat			

Total Calories	
Grams of Sugar	
Energy Level	
Attitude	

Workout:	Time:	Calories:

Date/Day _____ **Carb Level:** ❏High ❏Low ❏No ❏Free

Nutrient	Servings	Grams	%
Carbs			
Protein			
Fat			

Total Calories	
Grams of Sugar	
Energy Level	
Attitude	

Workout:	Time:	Calories:

Ending Weight:

Notes

Think about what went well this week,
look for small wins.

Week # _____

Starting Weight: _____

Date/Day _____ **Carb Level:** ❏High ❏Low ❏No ❏Free

Nutrient	Servings	Grams	%
Carbs			
Protein			
Fat			

Total Calories	
Grams of Sugar	
Energy Level	
Attitude	

Workout:	Time:	Calories:

Date/Day _____ **Carb Level:** ❏High ❏Low ❏No ❏Free

Nutrient	Servings	Grams	%
Carbs			
Protein			
Fat			

Total Calories	
Grams of Sugar	
Energy Level	
Attitude	

Workout:	Time:	Calories:

Date/Day _____ **Carb Level:** ❏High ❏Low ❏No ❏Free

Nutrient	Servings	Grams	%
Carbs			
Protein			
Fat			

Total Calories	
Grams of Sugar	
Energy Level	
Attitude	

Workout:	Time:	Calories:

Date/Day _____ **Carb Level:** ❏High ❏Low ❏No ❏Free

Nutrient	Servings	Grams	%
Carbs			
Protein			
Fat			

Total Calories	
Grams of Sugar	
Energy Level	
Attitude	

Workout:	Time:	Calories:

Date/Day _____ **Carb Level:** ❑High ❑Low ❑No ❑Free

Nutrient	Servings	Grams	%
Carbs			
Protein			
Fat			

Total Calories	
Grams of Sugar	
Energy Level	
Attitude	

Workout:	Time:	Calories:

Date/Day _____ **Carb Level:** ❑High ❑Low ❑No ❑Free

Nutrient	Servings	Grams	%
Carbs			
Protein			
Fat			

Total Calories	
Grams of Sugar	
Energy Level	
Attitude	

Workout:	Time:	Calories:

Date/Day _____ **Carb Level:** ❑High ❑Low ❑No ❑Free

Nutrient	Servings	Grams	%
Carbs			
Protein			
Fat			

Total Calories	
Grams of Sugar	
Energy Level	
Attitude	

Workout:	Time:	Calories:

Ending Weight:

Notes

Visualize yourself at your goal weight and play it over in your head each day.

Week # _____

Starting Weight: _____

Date/Day _____   **Carb Level:** ❑High ❑Low ❑No ❑Free

Nutrient	Servings	Grams	%
Carbs			
Protein			
Fat			

Total Calories	
Grams of Sugar	
Energy Level	
Attitude	

Workout:	Time:	Calories:

Date/Day _____   **Carb Level:** ❑High ❑Low ❑No ❑Free

Nutrient	Servings	Grams	%
Carbs			
Protein			
Fat			

Total Calories	
Grams of Sugar	
Energy Level	
Attitude	

Workout:	Time:	Calories:

Date/Day _____   **Carb Level:** ❑High ❑Low ❑No ❑Free

Nutrient	Servings	Grams	%
Carbs			
Protein			
Fat			

Total Calories	
Grams of Sugar	
Energy Level	
Attitude	

Workout:	Time:	Calories:

Date/Day _____   **Carb Level:** ❑High ❑Low ❑No ❑Free

Nutrient	Servings	Grams	%
Carbs			
Protein			
Fat			

Total Calories	
Grams of Sugar	
Energy Level	
Attitude	

Workout:	Time:	Calories:

Date/Day _____ **Carb Level:** ❑High ❑Low ❑No ❑Free

Nutrient	Servings	Grams	%
Carbs			
Protein			
Fat			

Total Calories	
Grams of Sugar	
Energy Level	
Attitude	

Workout:	Time:	Calories:

Date/Day _____ **Carb Level:** ❑High ❑Low ❑No ❑Free

Nutrient	Servings	Grams	%
Carbs			
Protein			
Fat			

Total Calories	
Grams of Sugar	
Energy Level	
Attitude	

Workout:	Time:	Calories:

Date/Day _____ **Carb Level:** ❑High ❑Low ❑No ❑Free

Nutrient	Servings	Grams	%
Carbs			
Protein			
Fat			

Total Calories	
Grams of Sugar	
Energy Level	
Attitude	

Workout:	Time:	Calories:

Ending Weight:

Notes

How much sugar are you eating each day? Can you reduce it?

Week # _____

Starting Weight: _____

Date/Day _____   **Carb Level:** ☐High ☐Low ☐No ☐Free

Nutrient	Servings	Grams	%
Carbs			
Protein			
Fat			

Total Calories	
Grams of Sugar	
Energy Level	
Attitude	

Workout:	Time:	Calories:

Date/Day _____   **Carb Level:** ☐High ☐Low ☐No ☐Free

Nutrient	Servings	Grams	%
Carbs			
Protein			
Fat			

Total Calories	
Grams of Sugar	
Energy Level	
Attitude	

Workout:	Time:	Calories:

Date/Day _____   **Carb Level:** ☐High ☐Low ☐No ☐Free

Nutrient	Servings	Grams	%
Carbs			
Protein			
Fat			

Total Calories	
Grams of Sugar	
Energy Level	
Attitude	

Workout:	Time:	Calories:

Date/Day _____   **Carb Level:** ☐High ☐Low ☐No ☐Free

Nutrient	Servings	Grams	%
Carbs			
Protein			
Fat			

Total Calories	
Grams of Sugar	
Energy Level	
Attitude	

Workout:	Time:	Calories:

Date/Day _____ Carb Level: ❑High ❑Low ❑No ❑Free

Nutrient	Servings	Grams	%
Carbs			
Protein			
Fat			

Total Calories	
Grams of Sugar	
Energy Level	
Attitude	

Workout:	Time:	Calories:

Date/Day _____ Carb Level: ❑High ❑Low ❑No ❑Free

Nutrient	Servings	Grams	%
Carbs			
Protein			
Fat			

Total Calories	
Grams of Sugar	
Energy Level	
Attitude	

Workout:	Time:	Calories:

Date/Day _____ Carb Level: ❑High ❑Low ❑No ❑Free

Nutrient	Servings	Grams	%
Carbs			
Protein			
Fat			

Total Calories	
Grams of Sugar	
Energy Level	
Attitude	

Workout:	Time:	Calories:

Ending Weight:

Notes

You are not alone in your challenge, reach out for help when you need it.

Week # _____

Starting Weight: _____

Date/Day _____ **Carb Level:** ❑High ❑Low ❑No ❑Free

Nutrient	Servings	Grams	%		
Carbs				Total Calories	
Protein				Grams of Sugar	
Fat				Energy Level	
				Attitude	

Workout:	Time:	Calories:

Date/Day _____ **Carb Level:** ❑High ❑Low ❑No ❑Free

Nutrient	Servings	Grams	%		
Carbs				Total Calories	
Protein				Grams of Sugar	
Fat				Energy Level	
				Attitude	

Workout:	Time:	Calories:

Date/Day _____ **Carb Level:** ❑High ❑Low ❑No ❑Free

Nutrient	Servings	Grams	%		
Carbs				Total Calories	
Protein				Grams of Sugar	
Fat				Energy Level	
				Attitude	

Workout:	Time:	Calories:

Date/Day _____ **Carb Level:** ❑High ❑Low ❑No ❑Free

Nutrient	Servings	Grams	%		
Carbs				Total Calories	
Protein				Grams of Sugar	
Fat				Energy Level	
				Attitude	

Workout:	Time:	Calories:

Date/Day _____ **Carb Level:** ❑**High** ❑**Low** ❑**No** ❑**Free**

Nutrient	Servings	Grams	%		Total Calories	
Carbs					Grams of Sugar	
Protein					Energy Level	
Fat					Attitude	

Workout:		Time:	Calories:

Date/Day _____ **Carb Level:** ❑**High** ❑**Low** ❑**No** ❑**Free**

Nutrient	Servings	Grams	%		Total Calories	
Carbs					Grams of Sugar	
Protein					Energy Level	
Fat					Attitude	

Workout:		Time:	Calories:

Date/Day _____ **Carb Level:** ❑**High** ❑**Low** ❑**No** ❑**Free**

Nutrient	Servings	Grams	%		Total Calories	
Carbs					Grams of Sugar	
Protein					Energy Level	
Fat					Attitude	

Workout:		Time:	Calories:

Ending Weight:

Notes

Energy levels starting to increase?

Week # _____

Starting Weight: _____

Date/Day _____   **Carb Level:** ❑High ❑Low ❑No ❑Free

Nutrient	Servings	Grams	%
Carbs			
Protein			
Fat			

Total Calories	
Grams of Sugar	
Energy Level	
Attitude	

Workout:	Time:	Calories:

Date/Day _____   **Carb Level:** ❑High ❑Low ❑No ❑Free

Nutrient	Servings	Grams	%
Carbs			
Protein			
Fat			

Total Calories	
Grams of Sugar	
Energy Level	
Attitude	

Workout:	Time:	Calories:

Date/Day _____   **Carb Level:** ❑High ❑Low ❑No ❑Free

Nutrient	Servings	Grams	%
Carbs			
Protein			
Fat			

Total Calories	
Grams of Sugar	
Energy Level	
Attitude	

Workout:	Time:	Calories:

Date/Day _____   **Carb Level:** ❑High ❑Low ❑No ❑Free

Nutrient	Servings	Grams	%
Carbs			
Protein			
Fat			

Total Calories	
Grams of Sugar	
Energy Level	
Attitude	

Workout:	Time:	Calories:

Date/Day _____ **Carb Level:** ❏High ❏Low ❏No ❏Free

Nutrient	Servings	Grams	%
Carbs			
Protein			
Fat			

Total Calories	
Grams of Sugar	
Energy Level	
Attitude	

Workout:	Time:	Calories:

Date/Day _____ **Carb Level:** ❏High ❏Low ❏No ❏Free

Nutrient	Servings	Grams	%
Carbs			
Protein			
Fat			

Total Calories	
Grams of Sugar	
Energy Level	
Attitude	

Workout:	Time:	Calories:

Date/Day _____ **Carb Level:** ❏High ❏Low ❏No ❏Free

Nutrient	Servings	Grams	%
Carbs			
Protein			
Fat			

Total Calories	
Grams of Sugar	
Energy Level	
Attitude	

Workout:	Time:	Calories:

Ending Weight:

Notes

What goals do you have for this week?

Week # _____

Starting Weight: _____

Date/Day _____ **Carb Level:** ❏High ❏Low ❏No ❏Free

Nutrient	Servings	Grams	%
Carbs			
Protein			
Fat			

Total Calories	
Grams of Sugar	
Energy Level	
Attitude	

Workout:	Time:	Calories:

Date/Day _____ **Carb Level:** ❏High ❏Low ❏No ❏Free

Nutrient	Servings	Grams	%
Carbs			
Protein			
Fat			

Total Calories	
Grams of Sugar	
Energy Level	
Attitude	

Workout:	Time:	Calories:

Date/Day _____ **Carb Level:** ❏High ❏Low ❏No ❏Free

Nutrient	Servings	Grams	%
Carbs			
Protein			
Fat			

Total Calories	
Grams of Sugar	
Energy Level	
Attitude	

Workout:	Time:	Calories:

Date/Day _____ **Carb Level:** ❏High ❏Low ❏No ❏Free

Nutrient	Servings	Grams	%
Carbs			
Protein			
Fat			

Total Calories	
Grams of Sugar	
Energy Level	
Attitude	

Workout:	Time:	Calories:

Date/Day_____ **Carb Level:** ❏High ❏Low ❏No ❏Free

Nutrient	Servings	Grams	%
Carbs			
Protein			
Fat			

Total Calories	
Grams of Sugar	
Energy Level	
Attitude	

Workout:	Time:	Calories:

Date/Day_____ **Carb Level:** ❏High ❏Low ❏No ❏Free

Nutrient	Servings	Grams	%
Carbs			
Protein			
Fat			

Total Calories	
Grams of Sugar	
Energy Level	
Attitude	

Workout:	Time:	Calories:

Date/Day_____ **Carb Level:** ❏High ❏Low ❏No ❏Free

Nutrient	Servings	Grams	%
Carbs			
Protein			
Fat			

Total Calories	
Grams of Sugar	
Energy Level	
Attitude	

Workout:	Time:	Calories:

Ending Weight:

Notes

Try a new exercise this week.

Week # _____

Starting Weight: _____

Date/Day _____   **Carb Level:** ❏High ❏Low ❏No ❏Free

Nutrient	Servings	Grams	%
Carbs			
Protein			
Fat			

Total Calories	
Grams of Sugar	
Energy Level	
Attitude	

Workout:	Time:	Calories:

Date/Day _____   **Carb Level:** ❏High ❏Low ❏No ❏Free

Nutrient	Servings	Grams	%
Carbs			
Protein			
Fat			

Total Calories	
Grams of Sugar	
Energy Level	
Attitude	

Workout:	Time:	Calories:

Date/Day _____   **Carb Level:** ❏High ❏Low ❏No ❏Free

Nutrient	Servings	Grams	%
Carbs			
Protein			
Fat			

Total Calories	
Grams of Sugar	
Energy Level	
Attitude	

Workout:	Time:	Calories:

Date/Day _____   **Carb Level:** ❏High ❏Low ❏No ❏Free

Nutrient	Servings	Grams	%
Carbs			
Protein			
Fat			

Total Calories	
Grams of Sugar	
Energy Level	
Attitude	

Workout:	Time:	Calories:

Date/Day _____ **Carb Level:** ❑**High** ❑**Low** ❑**No** ❑**Free**

Nutrient	Servings	Grams	%
Carbs			
Protein			
Fat			

Total Calories	
Grams of Sugar	
Energy Level	
Attitude	

Workout:	Time:	Calories:

Date/Day _____ **Carb Level:** ❑**High** ❑**Low** ❑**No** ❑**Free**

Nutrient	Servings	Grams	%
Carbs			
Protein			
Fat			

Total Calories	
Grams of Sugar	
Energy Level	
Attitude	

Workout:	Time:	Calories:

Date/Day _____ **Carb Level:** ❑**High** ❑**Low** ❑**No** ❑**Free**

Nutrient	Servings	Grams	%
Carbs			
Protein			
Fat			

Total Calories	
Grams of Sugar	
Energy Level	
Attitude	

Workout:	Time:	Calories:

Ending Weight:

Notes

If you don't give up, you won't have to start over.

Week # _____

Starting Weight: _____

Date/Day _____ **Carb Level:** ❏High ❏Low ❏No ❏Free

Nutrient	Servings	Grams	%		
Carbs				Total Calories	
Carbs				Grams of Sugar	
Protein				Energy Level	
Fat				Attitude	

Workout:	Time:	Calories:

Date/Day _____ **Carb Level:** ❏High ❏Low ❏No ❏Free

Nutrient	Servings	Grams	%		
Carbs				Total Calories	
Protein				Grams of Sugar	
Protein				Energy Level	
Fat				Attitude	

Workout:	Time:	Calories:

Date/Day _____ **Carb Level:** ❏High ❏Low ❏No ❏Free

Nutrient	Servings	Grams	%		
Carbs				Total Calories	
Protein				Grams of Sugar	
Protein				Energy Level	
Fat				Attitude	

Workout:	Time:	Calories:

Date/Day _____ **Carb Level:** ❏High ❏Low ❏No ❏Free

Nutrient	Servings	Grams	%		
Carbs				Total Calories	
Protein				Grams of Sugar	
Protein				Energy Level	
Fat				Attitude	

Workout:	Time:	Calories:

Date/Day _____ **Carb Level:** ❑**High** ❑**Low** ❑**No** ❑**Free**

Nutrient	Servings	Grams	%
Carbs			
Protein			
Fat			

Total Calories	
Grams of Sugar	
Energy Level	
Attitude	

Workout:	Time:	Calories:

Date/Day _____ **Carb Level:** ❑**High** ❑**Low** ❑**No** ❑**Free**

Nutrient	Servings	Grams	%
Carbs			
Protein			
Fat			

Total Calories	
Grams of Sugar	
Energy Level	
Attitude	

Workout:	Time:	Calories:

Date/Day _____ **Carb Level:** ❑**High** ❑**Low** ❑**No** ❑**Free**

Nutrient	Servings	Grams	%
Carbs			
Protein			
Fat			

Total Calories	
Grams of Sugar	
Energy Level	
Attitude	

Workout:	Time:	Calories:

Ending Weight:

Notes

Change just one small thing every week and you will change your life.

Week # _____

Starting Weight: _____

Date/Day _____ **Carb Level:** ❑High ❑Low ❑No ❑Free

Nutrient	Servings	Grams	%
Carbs			
Protein			
Fat			

Total Calories	
Grams of Sugar	
Energy Level	
Attitude	

Workout:	Time:	Calories:

Date/Day _____ **Carb Level:** ❑High ❑Low ❑No ❑Free

Nutrient	Servings	Grams	%
Carbs			
Protein			
Fat			

Total Calories	
Grams of Sugar	
Energy Level	
Attitude	

Workout:	Time:	Calories:

Date/Day _____ **Carb Level:** ❑High ❑Low ❑No ❑Free

Nutrient	Servings	Grams	%
Carbs			
Protein			
Fat			

Total Calories	
Grams of Sugar	
Energy Level	
Attitude	

Workout:	Time:	Calories:

Date/Day _____ **Carb Level:** ❑High ❑Low ❑No ❑Free

Nutrient	Servings	Grams	%
Carbs			
Protein			
Fat			

Total Calories	
Grams of Sugar	
Energy Level	
Attitude	

Workout:	Time:	Calories:

Date/Day_____   Carb Level: ❑High ❑Low ❑No ❑Free

Nutrient	Servings	Grams	%
Carbs			
Protein			
Fat			

Total Calories	
Grams of Sugar	
Energy Level	
Attitude	

Workout:	Time:	Calories:

Date/Day_____   Carb Level: ❑High ❑Low ❑No ❑Free

Nutrient	Servings	Grams	%
Carbs			
Protein			
Fat			

Total Calories	
Grams of Sugar	
Energy Level	
Attitude	

Workout:	Time:	Calories:

Date/Day_____   Carb Level: ❑High ❑Low ❑No ❑Free

Nutrient	Servings	Grams	%
Carbs			
Protein			
Fat			

Total Calories	
Grams of Sugar	
Energy Level	
Attitude	

Workout:	Time:	Calories:

Ending Weight:

Notes

You will never leave where you are until you decide where you want to be.

Week # _____

Starting Weight: _____

Date/Day _____ **Carb Level:** ❑High   ❑Low   ❑No   ❑Free

Nutrient	Servings	Grams	%
Carbs			
Protein			
Fat			

Total Calories	
Grams of Sugar	
Energy Level	
Attitude	

Workout:	Time:	Calories:

Date/Day _____ **Carb Level:** ❑High   ❑Low   ❑No   ❑Free

Nutrient	Servings	Grams	%
Carbs			
Protein			
Fat			

Total Calories	
Grams of Sugar	
Energy Level	
Attitude	

Workout:	Time:	Calories:

Date/Day _____ **Carb Level:** ❑High   ❑Low   ❑No   ❑Free

Nutrient	Servings	Grams	%
Carbs			
Protein			
Fat			

Total Calories	
Grams of Sugar	
Energy Level	
Attitude	

Workout:	Time:	Calories:

Date/Day _____ **Carb Level:** ❑High   ❑Low   ❑No   ❑Free

Nutrient	Servings	Grams	%
Carbs			
Protein			
Fat			

Total Calories	
Grams of Sugar	
Energy Level	
Attitude	

Workout:	Time:	Calories:

Date/Day_____ **Carb Level:** ❏High ❏Low ❏No ❏Free

Nutrient	Servings	Grams	%		Total Calories	
Carbs					Grams of Sugar	
Protein					Energy Level	
Fat					Attitude	

Workout:	Time:	Calories:

Date/Day_____ **Carb Level:** ❏High ❏Low ❏No ❏Free

Nutrient	Servings	Grams	%		Total Calories	
Carbs					Grams of Sugar	
Protein					Energy Level	
Fat					Attitude	

Workout:	Time:	Calories:

Date/Day_____ **Carb Level:** ❏High ❏Low ❏No ❏Free

Nutrient	Servings	Grams	%		Total Calories	
Carbs					Grams of Sugar	
Protein					Energy Level	
Fat					Attitude	

Workout:	Time:	Calories:

Ending Weight:

Notes

Stop wishing, start doing!

Week # _____

Starting Weight: _____

Date/Day _____   **Carb Level:** ❑High ❑Low ❑No ❑Free

Nutrient	Servings	Grams	%			
Carbs				Total Calories		
Protein				Grams of Sugar		
Fat				Energy Level		
				Attitude		

Workout:	Time:	Calories:

Date/Day _____   **Carb Level:** ❑High ❑Low ❑No ❑Free

Nutrient	Servings	Grams	%			
Carbs				Total Calories		
Protein				Grams of Sugar		
Fat				Energy Level		
				Attitude		

Workout:	Time:	Calories:

Date/Day _____   **Carb Level:** ❑High ❑Low ❑No ❑Free

Nutrient	Servings	Grams	%			
Carbs				Total Calories		
Protein				Grams of Sugar		
Fat				Energy Level		
				Attitude		

Workout:	Time:	Calories:

Date/Day _____   **Carb Level:** ❑High ❑Low ❑No ❑Free

Nutrient	Servings	Grams	%			
Carbs				Total Calories		
Protein				Grams of Sugar		
Fat				Energy Level		
				Attitude		

Workout:	Time:	Calories:

Date/Day_____ **Carb Level:** ❏High ❏Low ❏No ❏Free

Nutrient	Servings	Grams	%
Carbs			
Protein			
Fat			

Total Calories	
Grams of Sugar	
Energy Level	
Attitude	

Workout:	Time:	Calories:

Date/Day_____ **Carb Level:** ❏High ❏Low ❏No ❏Free

Nutrient	Servings	Grams	%
Carbs			
Protein			
Fat			

Total Calories	
Grams of Sugar	
Energy Level	
Attitude	

Workout:	Time:	Calories:

Date/Day_____ **Carb Level:** ❏High ❏Low ❏No ❏Free

Nutrient	Servings	Grams	%
Carbs			
Protein			
Fat			

Total Calories	
Grams of Sugar	
Energy Level	
Attitude	

Workout:	Time:	Calories:

Ending Weight:

Notes

What are you saying to yourself?
Positive self-talk makes a
difference.

Week # _____

Starting Weight: _____

Date/Day _____ **Carb Level:** ❑High ❑Low ❑No ❑Free

Nutrient	Servings	Grams	%
Carbs			
Protein			
Fat			

Total Calories	
Grams of Sugar	
Energy Level	
Attitude	

Workout:	Time:	Calories:

Date/Day _____ **Carb Level:** ❑High ❑Low ❑No ❑Free

Nutrient	Servings	Grams	%
Carbs			
Protein			
Fat			

Total Calories	
Grams of Sugar	
Energy Level	
Attitude	

Workout:	Time:	Calories:

Date/Day _____ **Carb Level:** ❑High ❑Low ❑No ❑Free

Nutrient	Servings	Grams	%
Carbs			
Protein			
Fat			

Total Calories	
Grams of Sugar	
Energy Level	
Attitude	

Workout:	Time:	Calories:

Date/Day _____ **Carb Level:** ❑High ❑Low ❑No ❑Free

Nutrient	Servings	Grams	%
Carbs			
Protein			
Fat			

Total Calories	
Grams of Sugar	
Energy Level	
Attitude	

Workout:	Time:	Calories:

Date/Day _____ Carb Level: ❏High ❏Low ❏No ❏Free

Nutrient	Servings	Grams	%
Carbs			
Protein			
Fat			

Total Calories	
Grams of Sugar	
Energy Level	
Attitude	

Workout:	Time:	Calories:

Date/Day _____ Carb Level: ❏High ❏Low ❏No ❏Free

Nutrient	Servings	Grams	%
Carbs			
Protein			
Fat			

Total Calories	
Grams of Sugar	
Energy Level	
Attitude	

Workout:	Time:	Calories:

Date/Day _____ Carb Level: ❏High ❏Low ❏No ❏Free

Nutrient	Servings	Grams	%
Carbs			
Protein			
Fat			

Total Calories	
Grams of Sugar	
Energy Level	
Attitude	

Workout:	Time:	Calories:

Ending Weight:

Notes

Focus on today, you can't change the past.

Week # _____

Starting Weight: _____

Date/Day _____ **Carb Level:** ❑High ❑Low ❑No ❑Free

Nutrient	Servings	Grams	%
Carbs			
Protein			
Fat			

Total Calories	
Grams of Sugar	
Energy Level	
Attitude	

Workout:	Time:	Calories:

Date/Day _____ **Carb Level:** ❑High ❑Low ❑No ❑Free

Nutrient	Servings	Grams	%
Carbs			
Protein			
Fat			

Total Calories	
Grams of Sugar	
Energy Level	
Attitude	

Workout:	Time:	Calories:

Date/Day _____ **Carb Level:** ❑High ❑Low ❑No ❑Free

Nutrient	Servings	Grams	%
Carbs			
Protein			
Fat			

Total Calories	
Grams of Sugar	
Energy Level	
Attitude	

Workout:	Time:	Calories:

Date/Day _____ **Carb Level:** ❑High ❑Low ❑No ❑Free

Nutrient	Servings	Grams	%
Carbs			
Protein			
Fat			

Total Calories	
Grams of Sugar	
Energy Level	
Attitude	

Workout:	Time:	Calories:

Date/Day _____ Carb Level: ❑High ❑Low ❑No ❑Free

Nutrient	Servings	Grams	%
Carbs			
Protein			
Fat			

Total Calories	
Grams of Sugar	
Energy Level	
Attitude	

Workout:	Time:	Calories:

Date/Day _____ Carb Level: ❑High ❑Low ❑No ❑Free

Nutrient	Servings	Grams	%
Carbs			
Protein			
Fat			

Total Calories	
Grams of Sugar	
Energy Level	
Attitude	

Workout:	Time:	Calories:

Date/Day _____ Carb Level: ❑High ❑Low ❑No ❑Free

Nutrient	Servings	Grams	%
Carbs			
Protein			
Fat			

Total Calories	
Grams of Sugar	
Energy Level	
Attitude	

Workout:	Time:	Calories:

Ending Weight:

Notes

Believe you can and you are
halfway there.

Week # _____

Starting Weight: _____

Date/Day _____ **Carb Level:** ❏High ❏Low ❏No ❏Free

Nutrient	Servings	Grams	%
Carbs			
Protein			
Fat			

Total Calories	
Grams of Sugar	
Energy Level	
Attitude	

Workout:	Time:	Calories:

Date/Day _____ **Carb Level:** ❏High ❏Low ❏No ❏Free

Nutrient	Servings	Grams	%
Carbs			
Protein			
Fat			

Total Calories	
Grams of Sugar	
Energy Level	
Attitude	

Workout:	Time:	Calories:

Date/Day _____ **Carb Level:** ❏High ❏Low ❏No ❏Free

Nutrient	Servings	Grams	%
Carbs			
Protein			
Fat			

Total Calories	
Grams of Sugar	
Energy Level	
Attitude	

Workout:	Time:	Calories:

Date/Day _____ **Carb Level:** ❏High ❏Low ❏No ❏Free

Nutrient	Servings	Grams	%
Carbs			
Protein			
Fat			

Total Calories	
Grams of Sugar	
Energy Level	
Attitude	

Workout:	Time:	Calories:

Date/Day _____ **Carb Level:** ❏High ❏Low ❏No ❏Free

Nutrient	Servings	Grams	%
Carbs			
Protein			
Fat			

Total Calories	
Grams of Sugar	
Energy Level	
Attitude	

Workout:	Time:	Calories:

Date/Day _____ **Carb Level:** ❏High ❏Low ❏No ❏Free

Nutrient	Servings	Grams	%
Carbs			
Protein			
Fat			

Total Calories	
Grams of Sugar	
Energy Level	
Attitude	

Workout:	Time:	Calories:

Date/Day _____ **Carb Level:** ❏High ❏Low ❏No ❏Free

Nutrient	Servings	Grams	%
Carbs			
Protein			
Fat			

Total Calories	
Grams of Sugar	
Energy Level	
Attitude	

Workout:	Time:	Calories:

Ending Weight:

Notes

If you don't take care of your body where will you live?

Week # _____

Starting Weight: _____

Date/Day _____ **Carb Level:** ❑High ❑Low ❑No ❑Free

Nutrient	Servings	Grams	%
Carbs			
Protein			
Fat			

Total Calories	
Grams of Sugar	
Energy Level	
Attitude	

Workout:	Time:	Calories:

Date/Day _____ **Carb Level:** ❑High ❑Low ❑No ❑Free

Nutrient	Servings	Grams	%
Carbs			
Protein			
Fat			

Total Calories	
Grams of Sugar	
Energy Level	
Attitude	

Workout:	Time:	Calories:

Date/Day _____ **Carb Level:** ❑High ❑Low ❑No ❑Free

Nutrient	Servings	Grams	%
Carbs			
Protein			
Fat			

Total Calories	
Grams of Sugar	
Energy Level	
Attitude	

Workout:	Time:	Calories:

Date/Day _____ **Carb Level:** ❑High ❑Low ❑No ❑Free

Nutrient	Servings	Grams	%
Carbs			
Protein			
Fat			

Total Calories	
Grams of Sugar	
Energy Level	
Attitude	

Workout:	Time:	Calories:

Date/Day_____ Carb Level: ❏High ❏Low ❏No ❏Free

Nutrient	Servings	Grams	%
Carbs			
Protein			
Fat			

Total Calories	
Grams of Sugar	
Energy Level	
Attitude	

Workout:	Time:	Calories:

Date/Day_____ Carb Level: ❏High ❏Low ❏No ❏Free

Nutrient	Servings	Grams	%
Carbs			
Protein			
Fat			

Total Calories	
Grams of Sugar	
Energy Level	
Attitude	

Workout:	Time:	Calories:

Date/Day_____ Carb Level: ❏High ❏Low ❏No ❏Free

Nutrient	Servings	Grams	%
Carbs			
Protein			
Fat			

Total Calories	
Grams of Sugar	
Energy Level	
Attitude	

Workout:	Time:	Calories:

Ending Weight:

Notes

Stop waiting for things to happen, go out and make them happen.

Week # _____

Starting Weight: _____

Date/Day _____   **Carb Level:** ❑High ❑Low ❑No ❑Free

Nutrient	Servings	Grams	%	Total Calories	
Carbs				Grams of Sugar	
Protein				Energy Level	
Fat				Attitude	

Workout:	Time:	Calories:

Date/Day _____   **Carb Level:** ❑High ❑Low ❑No ❑Free

Nutrient	Servings	Grams	%	Total Calories	
Carbs				Grams of Sugar	
Protein				Energy Level	
Fat				Attitude	

Workout:	Time:	Calories:

Date/Day _____   **Carb Level:** ❑High ❑Low ❑No ❑Free

Nutrient	Servings	Grams	%	Total Calories	
Carbs				Grams of Sugar	
Protein				Energy Level	
Fat				Attitude	

Workout:	Time:	Calories:

Date/Day _____   **Carb Level:** ❑High ❑Low ❑No ❑Free

Nutrient	Servings	Grams	%	Total Calories	
Carbs				Grams of Sugar	
Protein				Energy Level	
Fat				Attitude	

Workout:	Time:	Calories:

Date/Day _____ Carb Level: ❏High ❏Low ❏No ❏Free

Nutrient	Servings	Grams	%
Carbs			
Protein			
Fat			

Total Calories	
Grams of Sugar	
Energy Level	
Attitude	

Workout:	Time:	Calories:

Date/Day _____ Carb Level: ❏High ❏Low ❏No ❏Free

Nutrient	Servings	Grams	%
Carbs			
Protein			
Fat			

Total Calories	
Grams of Sugar	
Energy Level	
Attitude	

Workout:	Time:	Calories:

Date/Day _____ Carb Level: ❏High ❏Low ❏No ❏Free

Nutrient	Servings	Grams	%
Carbs			
Protein			
Fat			

Total Calories	
Grams of Sugar	
Energy Level	
Attitude	

Workout:	Time:	Calories:

Ending Weight:

Notes

Believe in yourself!

Week #_____

Starting Weight:_____

Date/Day_____ **Carb Level:** ❑High ❑Low ❑No ❑Free

Nutrient	Servings	Grams	%
Carbs			
Protein			
Fat			

Total Calories	
Grams of Sugar	
Energy Level	
Attitude	

Workout:	Time:	Calories:

Date/Day_____ **Carb Level:** ❑High ❑Low ❑No ❑Free

Nutrient	Servings	Grams	%
Carbs			
Protein			
Fat			

Total Calories	
Grams of Sugar	
Energy Level	
Attitude	

Workout:	Time:	Calories:

Date/Day_____ **Carb Level:** ❑High ❑Low ❑No ❑Free

Nutrient	Servings	Grams	%
Carbs			
Protein			
Fat			

Total Calories	
Grams of Sugar	
Energy Level	
Attitude	

Workout:	Time:	Calories:

Date/Day_____ **Carb Level:** ❑High ❑Low ❑No ❑Free

Nutrient	Servings	Grams	%
Carbs			
Protein			
Fat			

Total Calories	
Grams of Sugar	
Energy Level	
Attitude	

Workout:	Time:	Calories:

Date/Day_____ **Carb Level:** ❏High ❏Low ❏No ❏Free

Nutrient	Servings	Grams	%
Carbs			
Protein			
Fat			

Total Calories	
Grams of Sugar	
Energy Level	
Attitude	

Workout:	Time:	Calories:

Date/Day_____ **Carb Level:** ❏High ❏Low ❏No ❏Free

Nutrient	Servings	Grams	%
Carbs			
Protein			
Fat			

Total Calories	
Grams of Sugar	
Energy Level	
Attitude	

Workout:	Time:	Calories:

Date/Day_____ **Carb Level:** ❏High ❏Low ❏No ❏Free

Nutrient	Servings	Grams	%
Carbs			
Protein			
Fat			

Total Calories	
Grams of Sugar	
Energy Level	
Attitude	

Workout:	Time:	Calories:

Ending Weight:

Notes

Made in the USA
San Bernardino, CA
08 February 2016